Succeeding in Literature Reviews & Research Project Plans for Nursing Students

Succeeding in Literature Reviews & Research Project Plans for Nursing Students

5E

Graham R. Williamson
Andrew Whittaker

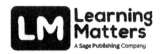

1 Oliver's Yard
55 City Road
London EC1Y 1SP

2455 Teller Road
Thousand Oaks
California 91320

Unit No 323-333, Third Floor, F-Block
International Trade Tower
Nehru Place, New Delhi – 110 019

8 Marina View Suite 43-053
Asia Square Tower 1
Singapore 018960

Editor: Martha Cunneen
Development editor: Richenda Milton-Daws
Senior project editor: Chris Marke
Project management: Westchester Publishing
Marketing manager: Ruslana Khatagova
Cover design: Sheila Tong
Typeset by: C&M Digitals (P) Ltd, Chennai, India
Printed and bound by CPI Group (UK) Ltd, Croydon, CR0 4YY

Library of Congress Control Number: 2024944293

British Library Cataloguing in Publication Data

A catalogue record for this book is available from the British Library

ISBN 978-1-5297-7982-0
ISBN 978-1-5297-7981-3 (Pbk)

Contents

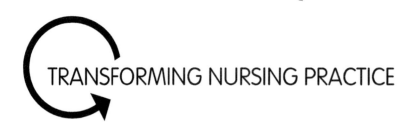

TRANSFORMING NURSING PRACTICE

Transforming Nursing Practice is a series tailor made for pre-registration student nurses. Each book in the series is:

 Affordable

 Full of active learning features

 Mapped to the NMC Standards of proficiency for registered nurses

 Focused on applying theory to practice

Each book addresses a core topic and they have been carefully developed to be simple to use, quick to read and written in clear language.

An invaluable series of books that explicitly relates to the NMC standards. Each book covers a different topic that students need to explore in order to develop into a qualified nurse... I would recommend this series to all Pre-Registered nursing students whatever their field or year of study.

LINDA ROBSON,
Senior Lecturer at Edge Hill University

Many titles in the series are on our recommended reading list and for good reason - the content is up to date and easy to read. These are the books that actually get used beyond training and into your nursing career.

EMMA LYDON,
Adult Student Nursing

ABOUT THE SERIES EDITORS

DR MOOI STANDING is an Independent Nursing Consultant (UK and International) and is responsible for the core knowledge, adult nursing and personal and professional learning skills titles. She is an experienced NMC Quality Assurance Reviewer of educational programmes and a Professional Regulator Panellist on the NMC Practice Committee. Mooi is also Board member of Special Olympics Malaysia, enabling people with intellectual disabilities to participate in sports and athletics nationally and internationally.

DR SANDRA WALKER is a Clinical Academic in Mental Health working between Southern Health Trust and the University of Southampton and responsible for the mental health nursing titles. She is a Qualified Mental Health Nurse with a wide range of clinical experience spanning more than 25 years.

BESTSELLING TEXTBOOKS

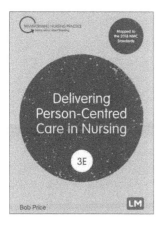

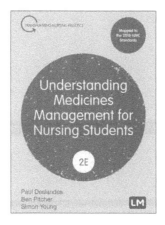

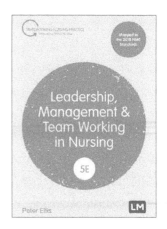

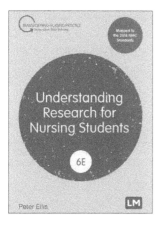

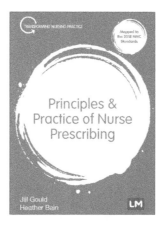

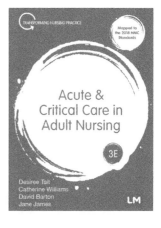

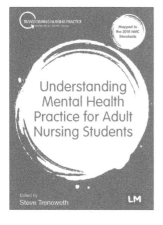

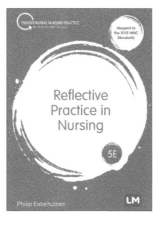

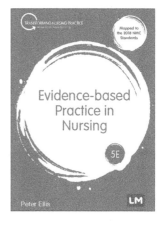

You can find a full list of textbooks in the *Transforming Nursing Practice* series at
https://uk.sagepub.com/TNP-series

About the authors

Dr Graham R. Williamson is an Associate Professor in Adult Nursing at the University of Plymouth School of Nursing and Midwifery, based at the Exeter School of Nursing. His clinical background is in acute medical nursing. His areas of teaching expertise are in evidence-based practice and research. His research interests concern supporting students in clinical practice, latterly in regard to Collaborative Learning in Practice.

Dr Andrew Whittaker is Emeritus Professor in Health and Social Care Research at London South Bank University. He has taught nursing students since the early 1990s and teaches research skills to undergraduate and postgraduate students. His research interests focus upon decision making and the nature of expertise in health and social care settings. He has worked in adult and child mental health and was the director of a mental health voluntary organisation.

Foreword

Succeeding in Literature Reviews and Research Project Plans for Nursing Students enables readers to prepare for, organise, carry out and successfully complete a comprehensive literature review or research proposal. Hence, reading this book will help nursing students to develop and apply key analytical and critical graduate skills needed to qualify as registered nurses. It is therefore an essential book for all undergraduate pre-registration nursing students. The authors are very experienced in teaching, supporting and supervising nursing students who are undertaking a literature review or research project, and the writing style of the book reflects this. They recognise that this final-year assignment/dissertation is likely to be the most demanding academic piece of work that students have to produce in becoming graduate nurses. Readers are encouraged to actively participate as they are guided through choosing a nursing topic, developing questions about it, accessing and critically reviewing research literature, considering ethical issues, proposing research, where applicable, and writing up their literature review or research proposal. Case studies are used throughout the book, linking theory to practice and highlighting how research studies generate knowledge for nurses to apply in delivering safe, effective, evidence-based and ethical care to their patients.

In the fifth edition of this invaluable book the authors have updated references and websites with additional learning resources and added new input on clinical practice development and quality improvement initiatives. The revisions reinforce the book's established strengths (recognised by nursing students and nurse educators) in systematically guiding readers to succeed in their final-year assignment/dissertation, be it a literature review or a research proposal. The authors emphasise the transferability of such analytical and critical skills in addressing both *Future Nurse: Standards of Proficiency for Registered Nurses* (NMC, 2018a), and the knowledge and skills NHS employers require nurses to possess, such as leadership, communication and service development/quality improvement. These analytical and critical skills are also essential for registered nurses to demonstrate in relation to *The Code: Professional Standards of Practice and Behaviour for Nurses, Midwives and Nursing Associates* (NMC, 2018b). For example, Item 6: *Always practise in line with the best available evidence;* and Item 25: *Provide leadership to make sure people's wellbeing is protected and to improve their experiences of the health and care system.*

Dr. Mooi Standing, Series Editor

Acknowledgements

Graham Williamson would like to dedicate this book to the thousands of students who have undertaken modules related to this subject area at the University of Plymouth over the years. It is a pleasure to see the high standards achieved by those who work hard at this. It is also a pleasure to meet ex-students years later as registrants.

Andrew Whittaker would like to dedicate this book to his much-loved father, Ian Whittaker (1931–2023). He would like to thank his supportive former colleagues at London South Bank University, particularly Tirion Havard, Hiten Solanki, Andrea Colquhoun, Michelle Evans and Martyn Higgins. He has appreciated the support of staff at Learning Matters at Sage, particularly Martha Cunneen and Ruth Lilly, who have been helpful and encouraging. He would like to thank current and past students for their helpful comments and suggestions.

Andrew would also like to thank his mother Christine, sister Sally, Joe, Lauren-Kate and Ben for their support and encouragement. He would like to thank his stepmother Vivien, Rebecca, Samantha and Lily and, most of all, he would like to thank his wife, Christina, for her love and support.

Artwork

The authors and publisher are grateful for permissions to reproduce the following artwork:

> **Figure 6.1: CONSORT 2010 flow diagram**. Reproduced from Moher et al. (2010). Made available under the Wikimedia Creative Commons License via Wikipedia (see http://creativecommons.org/licenses/by/3.0 for terms and conditions).

> **Figure 7.1: Normal distribution curve**. Adapted from an original graph by Jeremy Kemp (2 September 2005). Made available under the Wikimedia Creative Commons License via Wikipedia (see http://creativecommons.org/licenses/by-sa/3.0 for terms and conditions).

> **Figure 7.4: Confidence intervals containing point estimates**. Adapted from an original graph by Sigbert (8 December 2008). Made available under the Wikimedia Creative Commons License via Wikipedia (see http://creativecommons.org/licenses/by-sa/3.0 for terms and conditions).

Figure 7.5: Scatterplot showing a strong positive correlation between age and wrinkles. Adapted from an original graph by Lars Aronsson (8 December 2008). Made available under the Wikimedia Creative Commons License via Wikipedia (see http://creativecommons.org/licenses/by-sa/3.0 for terms and conditions).

Figure 7.6: Forest plot showing confidence intervals, point estimates as black boxes and a summary measure in the larger diamond. Reproduced from an original graph by Jimjamjak (4 May 2010). Made available under the Wikimedia Creative Commons License via Wikipedia (see http://creativecommons.org/licenses/by-sa/3.0/deed.en for terms and conditions). Under the terms of the GNU licence the original must be made available to readers and this is available at http://upload.wikimedia.org/wikipedia/commons/f/f0/Generic_forest_plot.png.

Figure 8.1: Generic funnel plot. Reproduced from an original graph by Nousernamesleft (21 January 2008). Made freely available for any purpose under the Wikimedia Creative Commons License via Wikipedia (see http://commons.wikimedia.org/wiki/Main_Page for further information).

Figure 8.2: Funnel plot showing publication bias. Adapted from an original graph by Nousernamesleft (21 January 2008). Made freely available for any purpose under the Wikimedia Creative Commons License via Wikipedia (see http://commons.wikimedia.org/wiki/Main_Page for further information).

Figure 8.3: The Cochrane Collaboration logo. Used with permission from Nick Royle, CEO, the Cochrane Collaboration, Oxford, UK. The Cochrane Collaboration logo is a registered trademark of the Cochrane Collaboration.

Figure 11.1: Gantt chart for project planning. Adapted from an original diagram by Garry L. Booker (8 October 2007) and released into the public domain via Wikipedia. Made available under the Wikimedia Creative Commons License via Wikipedia (see http://creativecommons.org/licenses/by-sa/3.0/deed.en for terms and conditions).

Every effort has been made to trace all copyright holders within the book, but if any have been inadvertently overlooked the publisher will be pleased to make the necessary arrangements at the first opportunity.

Introduction

This book is written for students of nursing who are developing the knowledge and skills to complete the research project plans and literature reviews which are increasingly components of their programmes, typically as third-year studies. While it is primarily aimed at students in their final year or level of study on an undergraduate degree, it will also be useful for students on postgraduate programmes with a research component, including those studying at master's level. It would also assist students undertaking a range of social and healthcare courses in further education, including social workers, midwives, occupational therapists and other health and social care professionals for whom research, project planning and reviewing literature are essential elements. Experienced and qualified nurses, especially those undertaking postgraduate studies, will also be able to use this book for consultation, teaching and revision and to gain an insight into the expectations raised in nursing degree programmes.

Requirements for nurse education

Nurse education has undergone a major transformation over the last 30 years as programmes of study have moved into university settings. After a consultation process that began in summer 2017 and was completed with the Nursing and Midwifery Council (NMC) approval on 28 March 2018, the NMC introduced new standards for nurses and this book has been revised to reflect them. All the NMC standards can be accessed via the NMC website, and we cite *Future Nurse: Standards of Proficiency for Registered Nurses* (NMC, 2018a). We refer extensively below to these NMC and the Quality Assurance Agency (QAA) requirements to illustrate the extent to which the NMC as a professional regulatory body, and the QAA as the agency that reviews the quality and standards of higher education in universities, insist that nurses develop research and evidence-based practice skills. Taken as a whole, this book maps to these standards.

NMC Future Nurse: Standards of Proficiency for Registered Nurses

The NMC (2018a) *Future Nurse: Standards of Proficiency for Registered Nurses* indicates the proficiencies expected for nurses at the point of registration, and continually emphasises the need for good understanding of research and the evidence base for practice. Nurses need the confidence and ability to think critically, apply knowledge and skills, and provide

(Continued)

(Continued)

expert, evidence-based, direct nursing care as the centre of all registered nursing practice (NMC, 2018a). The NMC (2018a, page 38) definition of evidence-based, person-centred nursing care is that nurses are required to make sure that any care and treatment is given to people based on what research has shown to be most effective. The judgement and experience of the nurse and the views of the person should also be taken into account when choosing which treatment is most likely to be successful for an individual.

The following sections are the specific references to research and evidence, adapted from the documents.

Platform 1: Being an accountable professional

Registered nurses act in the best interests of people, putting them first and providing nursing care that is person-centred, safe and compassionate. They act professionally at all times and use their knowledge and experience to make evidence-based decisions about care. They communicate effectively, are role models for others, and are accountable for their actions. Registered nurses continually reflect on their practice and keep abreast of new and emerging developments in nursing, health and care.

Outcomes
At the point of registration, the registered nurse will be able to:

1.7 Demonstrate an understanding of research methods, ethics and governance in order to critically analyse, safely use, share and apply research findings to promote and inform best nursing practice.
1.8 Demonstrate the knowledge, skills and ability to think critically when applying evidence and drawing on experience to make evidence-informed decisions in all situations.
1.20 Safely demonstrate evidence-based practice in all skills and procedures.

Platform 2: Promoting health and preventing ill health

Registered nurses play a key role in improving and maintaining the mental, physical and behavioural health and well-being of people, families, communities and populations. They support and enable people at all stages of life and in all care settings to make informed choices about how to manage health challenges in order to maximise their quality of life and improve health outcomes. They are actively involved in the prevention of and protection against disease and ill health and engage in public health, community development and global health agendas, and in the reduction of health inequalities.

Outcomes
At the point of registration, the registered nurse will be able to:

2.5 Promote and improve mental, physical, behavioural and other health-related outcomes by understanding and explaining the principles, practice and evidence-base for health screening programmes.

2.11 Promote health and prevent ill health by understanding and explaining to people the principles of pathogenesis, immunology and the evidence-base for immunisation, vaccination and herd immunity.

Platform 3: Assessing needs and planning care

Registered nurses prioritise the needs of people when assessing and reviewing their mental, physical, cognitive, behavioural, social and spiritual needs. They use information obtained during assessments to identify the priorities and requirements for person-centred and evidence-based nursing interventions and support. They work in partnership with people to develop person-centred care plans that take into account their circumstances, characteristics and preferences.

Outcomes
At the point of registration, the registered nurse will be able to:

3.5 Demonstrate the ability to accurately process all information gathered during the assessment process to identify needs for individualised nursing care and develop person-centred evidence-based plans for nursing interventions with agreed goals.

Platform 4: Providing and evaluating care

Registered nurses take the lead in providing evidence-based, compassionate and safe nursing interventions. They ensure that care they provide and delegate is person-centred and of a consistently high standard. They support people of all ages in a range of care settings. They work in partnership with people, families and carers to evaluate whether care is effective and that the goals of care have been met in line with their wishes, preferences and desired outcomes.

Outcomes
At the point of registration, the registered nurse will be able to:

4.1 Demonstrate and apply an understanding of what is important to people and how to use this knowledge to ensure their needs for safety, dignity, privacy, comfort and sleep can be met, acting as a role model for others in providing evidence-based person-centred care.

4.6 Demonstrate the knowledge, skills and ability to act as a role model for others in providing evidence-based nursing care to meet people's needs related to nutrition, hydration and bladder and bowel health.

4.7 Demonstrate the knowledge, skills and ability to act as a role model for others in providing evidence-based, person-centred nursing care to meet people's needs related to mobility, hygiene, oral care, wound care and skin integrity.

4.9 Demonstrate the knowledge and skills required to prioritise what is important to people and their families when providing evidence-based person-centred nursing care at

(Continued)

(Continued)

      end of life including the care of people who are dying, families, the deceased and the bereaved.

4.12 Demonstrate the ability to manage commonly encountered devices and confidently carry out related nursing procedures to meet people's needs for evidence-based, person-centred care.

In addition to the specific requirements above, the NMC (2018a) standards contain a number of skills for which the NMC requires an awareness of evidence to support best practice in compassionate, evidence-based person-centred nursing care, in each field. These are as outlined in Annexe A: Communication and relationship management skills and Annexe B: Nursing procedures.

Benchmark Statement for Health Care Programmes

The QAA (2001) Benchmark Statement for Health Care Programmes indicates that in nursing the following are important in relation to research and evidence.

A1 Professional autonomy and accountability

The award holder should be able to:

- contribute to the development and dissemination of evidence-based practice within professional contexts.

A4 Profession and employer context

The award holder should be able to:

- recognise the value of research and other scholarly activity in relation to the development of the profession and of patient/client care;
- recognise the need for changes in practice from best available evidence.

The study of nursing encompasses the following principle:

- the application of current knowledge and research to nursing practice across the health and illness continuum.

B2 Formulation of plans and strategies for meeting healthcare needs

The award holder should be able to:

- use evidence-based options to facilitate patient choice and inform nursing interventions.

B3 Practice

The award holder should be able to:

- conduct appropriate activities skilfully and in accordance with best/evidence-based practice;
- apply evidence-based knowledge to inform nursing care decisions.

C1 Knowledge and understanding

The award holder should be able to demonstrate:

- understanding of the key concepts of the disciplines that underpin the education and training of all healthcare professionals, and detailed knowledge of some of these. The latter would include a broad understanding of:
  - o health and social care philosophy and policy, and its translation into ethical and evidence-based practice.

C2 Associated skills

The award holder should be able to:

Information gathering

- seek out research-based evidence related to specific client groups;
- show an ability to gather and evaluate evidence and information from a wide range of sources;
- show an ability to use methods of enquiry to collect and interpret data in order to provide information that would inform or benefit practice.

Problem solving and data collection and interpretation

- analyse, interpret and assess the value of evidence to inform problem solving.

Information technology

- access healthcare research and literature databases.

Teaching, learning and assessment
Generic and enabling skills

Programmes should be designed to facilitate students' acquisition of effective communication skills, team working, problem solving, the use of IT, research methodology and critical reasoning.

B Principles and concepts: application

The award holder should be able to:

- demonstrate critical understanding of research-based knowledge and the application to practice;

(Continued)

5

(Continued)

- use relevant theoretical and research evidence to inform a comprehensive, systematic assessment of the physical, psychological, social and spiritual needs of patients, clients and communities;
- critically evaluate research findings and suggest changes to planned care;
- use appropriate research and other evidence to underpin nursing decisions that can be justified, even when made on the basis of limited information.

C Subject knowledge, understanding and associated skills

The award holder should be able to:

- demonstrate an understanding of research and other evidence and, where appropriate, apply findings to practice;
- critically evaluate research findings, suggest changes to practice and contribute to healthcare research to inform practice development.

Implications for students

Although nursing is a very practical occupation, this emphasis can be mistaken as a call for 'common sense' rather than 'book knowledge'. However, common sense can be used to justify a range of taken-for-granted assumptions that are often unspoken and can perpetuate poor practice when they go unchallenged. Instead, an internationally accepted development in healthcare decision making is to maintain a patient focus and integrate the best of research findings, theoretical and experiential knowledge to ensure care is based on up-to-date evidence and is appropriate for the patient's/ service user's needs. You will find this referred to as evidence-informed decision making, indicating how important evidence should be in the treatment and care of individual patients and clients. This approach is known as clinical effectiveness, and relies on evidence-based practice to ensure that research findings are robust, but also that their application takes into account the needs and wishes of the patient/ client and the experience of the practitioner. This book concentrates on supporting you to develop the core skills required to complete the research-project-planning and literature-reviewing components of your programmes, particularly at degree level. An action-oriented approach helps to facilitate evaluation and review of your practice. Case studies, reflecting a range of different practice settings, will be used throughout to enhance this process and to illustrate key points.

Book structure

This book contains four sections, with 11 chapters. Section 1 is called *Getting started*, and contains one large chapter called *Getting started on your final-year project*. It provides an overview of literature reviews, project plans and dissertations, including useful information about why they are undertaken, some of the expectations that go along with them, and what they can give you in terms of transferable skills and benefits in practice. This chapter also looks at the role of research in your final-year project.

Section 2 is called *Planning and preparing for your final-year project*, and contains two chapters. Chapter 2 is *Planning and undertaking a literature review*, which focuses on the 'how to' aspects of this, as well as offering some insights, which will help you to appraise and use research to inform practice. Chapter 3 is *Planning your research proposal or dissertation* and, again, provides practical material on how this can best be achieved.

In Section 3, *Using and critiquing research for your final-year project*, there are six chapters, and these have been written with the emphasis on helping students decide which approaches to use as part of their research plans or proposals, with some insights into how different approaches might be assessed as part of a literature review. There is little on undertaking the methods *per se*; instead, the emphasis is on understanding them, with a focus on the 'how' and 'why' rather than the 'what'. The first chapter of Section 3, *Using and critiquing qualitative research methods: interviews and focus groups* (Chapter 4), contains material on interviews and focus groups. Chapter 5 contains material on *Analysing qualitative data*, and looks at a popular method called thematic analysis. Chapter 6, *Using and critiquing research methods: surveys and experimental designs*, has a focus on experimental designs and randomised controlled trials, as well as surveys. Chapter 7, *Analysing quantitative data and understanding basic statistics*, provides some introductory ideas on quantitative research methods of data analysis. Chapter 8, *Using and critiquing systematic reviews and meta-analyses*, presents some details on how students can plan a protocol for a systematic review as well as introducing some basic concepts in this area for qualitative, quantitative and mixed-methods reviews. Finally, Chapter 9 looks at the important issue of *Translating evidence into practice*.

The last section is Section 4: *Writing and finishing*. This section will help you produce an acceptable finished product for your work. Chapter 10 is called *Writing up your literature review*, and Chapter 11 looks at issues in *Writing your research proposal and dissertation*.

Concluding remarks are offered at the end of the book.

Learning features

The book is interactive. You are encouraged to work through it as an active participant, taking responsibility for your learning, in order to increase your knowledge, understanding and ability to apply this learning to practice.

Case studies throughout the book will help you to examine the theoretical material discussed in the context of nursing practice. We have devised activities that require you to reflect on experiences, situations and events and help you to review and summarise learning undertaken. In this way, your knowledge will become deeply embedded as part of your development. When you come to apply your learning in practice, the reflection undertaken here will help you to understand the relevance of research concepts to practice.

This book will introduce knowledge and learning activities for you as a student nurse concerning the central processes relating to research in all areas of the discipline. Suggestions for further reading are made at the end of each chapter.

Section 1

Getting started

Chapter 1 Getting started on your final-year project

Chapter aims

After reading this chapter, you should have developed an understanding of these areas:

- nursing and research;
- an overview of literature reviews, project plans and dissertations;
- key terms in research;
- an introduction to quantitative and qualitative research paradigms and mixed-methods approaches;
- research designs from particular traditions (including action research, evaluation research, participatory and emancipatory research, case studies);
- research attitude.

Introduction

You are about to embark upon a process that is likely to change the way you think. You will gain tools for challenging your own thinking and the thinking of others and get a glimpse 'behind the scenes' at how knowledge is created. As a result, you are likely to experience more freedom than with any other part of the course for intensive study of a topic that interests you.

Historically, nursing has seen itself as a 'practical' subject and has drawn upon other disciplines to provide a research base to inform its interventions. Medicine, sociology, psychology and biology have been the disciplines that have been the most influential; all of these have relatively well-established research bases. As nursing has evolved as a discipline and is now an all-graduate profession at NHS Band 5, there has been a shift towards developing nursing's own research base.

The use of evidence to inform professional nursing practice (as opposed to looking after people based on custom-and-practice or tradition) is now widely established as essential (Ellis, 2023). Thus developing an understanding of research and related concepts, such as literature searching and ethics, is an important part of the pre-registration nursing degree, usually occurring in the later course years. So you will have become accustomed to traditional academic writing and competence-based assessments such as placement portfolios; however, the prospect of learning a new vocabulary and set of skills can be a little daunting. For example, although all students must demonstrate numerical proficiency before qualifying, this may not translate into confidence in critically appraising statistical information. Even the language of research design, methodology and data analysis can seem technical and remote from students' experiences.

Activity 1.1   Reflection

Take a sheet of blank paper. Think of the term 'research' and jot down any ideas that occur to you.

Take a separate sheet of paper and jot down the emotions provoked by the idea of engaging in research.

As this is a personal reflective activity, there is no outline answer at the end of the chapter.

Some students find that a lot of negative emotions are forthcoming. Reinforcing negative emotions by going over them repeatedly will not help you to overcome them. It is very important that these are supplanted by some positives, so try the following: visualise yourself successfully completing your dissertation or module assignment, handing it in and getting a really good mark. How good would that feel? Next, think about how much you want to be a nurse – hopefully quite a lot at this stage of your programme. This is one module or assignment that is between you and your goal of becoming a nurse, but it is achievable; thousands of students do something similar every year. Visualise yourself at your graduation, in your best clothes, with your friends and family clapping as you receive your certificate. Return to this imagery if things get tough when you are writing. You now have a positive goal in sight rather than negative emotions, and successfully completing your dissertation is just part of that.

For many nurses, 'research' is something that is either intimidating or boring – perhaps both. It is done by other people, such as psychologists or doctors, using highly complex and technical procedures. We hope to challenge these myths throughout this book and demonstrate to you that research is something that can be interesting and straightforward. For nurses, the point of research is not as a purely academic exercise but rather about how it contributes to improvements in everyday nursing practice and patient care. This is reflected in the NMC *Standards for Pre-registration Nursing Education* (NMC,

2018a) as well as the QAA's (QAA, 2001) subject benchmarks for nursing, listed in the Introduction. This is because nurse education prepares students to attain increasing levels of professional competence throughout the degree programme, culminating in their readiness to become registered nurses, once they have fulfilled the requirements of *The Code* (NMC, 2018b). While few nursing students will undertake a piece of research as a final-year project, many will be asked to undertake a *literature review*, often in conjunction with a research proposal. This book therefore focuses on these aspects: it is about understanding and doing literature reviews and applying research concepts to proposal writing, rather than about research per se.

The purpose of such extended pieces of work is that they provide an opportunity to explore and develop key, transferable academic skills such as project management, analysis and synthesis, and critiquing and developing a deeper understanding of research and evidence to underpin practice.

By reviewing the literature in an area, you will also gain in-depth knowledge of a topic that you are interested in from the practice setting. As an overview, undertaking a literature review involves an exhaustive search and retrieval exercise using a systematic process of:

- searching electronic databases using key words;
- specifying criteria for the retrieval of articles from the search;
- using critical appraisal to examine the articles' strengths and weaknesses, usually against some agreed criteria;
- synthesis of the literature to uncover some insights (possibly new ones) as evidenced by this body of knowledge.

An important development in nursing and healthcare in this field is that of systematic reviews and meta-analyses. This usually applies to quantitative work, although there are qualitative, narrative approaches to it. We explore these concepts more fully in Chapter 8.

Writing a project proposal will be useful and you will gain from the experience because, as well as requiring you to understand research concepts more fully and plan a coherent study, it may inform future studies such as a master's degree. You will also be addressing the professional standards listed in the Introduction and these in turn will influence your patient care when you are qualified.

Research project proposals need to include a summary of the literature on the topic you have chosen. This summary may or may not need to be sourced in a systematic review, but it will need to contain a background and rationale for the proposal and some idea about how the existing literature informs your study. You will need to have a research question, a sentence with a question mark at the end, as well as aims and objectives. Ensure that these are achievable and not too ambitious. You will probably be asked to write about your underlying approach, whether qualitative or quantitative. You would then develop an outline of how you intend to conduct the study, indicating what methods of data collection and analysis you will use (this is why we spend time below outlining some of the different ways in which this can be understood), as well as a time-table, resources and plan for dissemination of the findings.

'Dissertation' is a term that is applied to some form of extended study, usually under-taken as part of an academic award. For our purposes, it can denote a third-year piece of work, with an element of choice involved. Dissertations do not usually take an essay format, in which students are asked to answer a question; rather, they require students to choose an area of practice of their own interest and explore that in some way. A dissertation would normally have some element of research in it, and the term is most frequently associated with a research project where data collection and analysis are carried out, although this is not common in nursing courses. In nursing, a dissertation could be a project where literature is reviewed, and conclusions and recommendations drawn and may include a research proposal. You may not even have a 'dissertation module'; if you do have one, be careful to write it following the structure requirements given at your institution. As it is usually worth more than the normal number of credits it is perhaps 5,000 words or longer, and will involve an element of critical appraisal, analysis and synthesis.

Transferable skills

Completing your project will provide you with the following range of transferable skills:

- project management skills, from first conception through to completion. These include time management and planning skills, as well as evaluation and implementation skills;
- the ability to find and begin to critically evaluate research studies, rather than accepting them at face value. This can lead to increased confidence to question your own practice and the practice of others;
- the ability to think and study independently and take responsibility for your own learning as an autonomous practitioner. This can lead to increased curiosity and openness to new ideas.

These are all essential skills that will increase your employability and positively improve your practice.

Professional development and reflective practice

Great emphasis is placed on developing skills of reflection about, in and on practice. This has developed over many years in nursing. It is important also that you reflect on practice.

Developing a questioning approach that looks in a critical way at how you approach the research task and seeks to heighten your skills will help you to refine your practice and deepen your understanding of research concepts. Reflection is central to good nursing practice, but only if action results from that reflection.

Reflecting about, in and on your practice is not only important during your nurse preparation programme; it is considered key to continuing professional development. As we move to a profession that acknowledges lifelong learning as a way of keeping up to date, ensuring that research informs practice and honing skills and values for practice, it is important to begin the process at the outset of your development. This is reinforced by the professional standards discussed in the Introduction.

The role of research in your projects

We will now look over the key terms and approaches in research, some of which you may have come across before, to help you recall these prior to starting your project. Although you may not be working with all these methods within your course, you will need to be familiar with them, and their application in nursing, in order to complete a research proposal or plan, and to assess literature as part of your literature review.

Future chapters will look at each of these in more detail to enable you to select the most appropriate methods for your research proposal. So, consider the notes below as a 'refresher', which we will then go on to cover in more detail and relate more closely to study design. We have begun by asking you to reflect upon your initial thoughts about engaging in research. Below, you will be introduced to key terms. The distinction between quantitative and qualitative approaches will be discussed. You will be asked to consider a range of research designs from particular traditions to illustrate the wide diversity of approaches.

Key terms in research

As with any new area of study, you need to understand new terminology that can seem technical and confusing. Here are a few key terms that you will come across when studying for, and considering the design of, your research proposal or project. There is considerable debate about the exact use of specific terms, but the definitions below are generally agreed upon and are the meanings that are used in this book.

Data refers to the information that you are going to collect in order to answer your research question; for example, the words used by your interview participants or numerical information from your questionnaires. Strictly speaking, data is a plural rather than a singular noun (the singular is 'datum') and this convention will be kept throughout this book.

Epistemology is the study of knowledge and addresses the question of what counts as legitimate knowledge. Research projects contain assumptions about what is legitimate knowledge, and this is known as its *epistemological position* or *stance*.

Methodology refers to the totality of how you are going to undertake your research. It includes the research approach (or study design) that you will use, including your epistemological position and the specific research methods you will choose, such as interviews or questionnaires.

Research approach or paradigm refers to the traditional division between quantitative and qualitative traditions in research, which will be discussed further in this chapter.

Research method refers to the practical way in which you are going to collect your data. Commonly used methods in healthcare research are interviews, questionnaires, *focus groups* and rating scales.

Sampling refers to the process of selecting the participants (or other data sources, e.g. documents) that will be involved in your study. Your *sample* (the selection of people or other data sources) is chosen from the total possible data sources, known as the *population*.

Research participants replaces the outmoded term 'research subjects', because the latter term suggests that people involved in research should have a passive role in a process to which they are 'subjected'. The term 'participants' suggests a more active and equal role, in which participation is informed and freely chosen.

Quantitative research tends to emphasise quantification and measurement, which can be analysed using statistical tests to establish a relationship between variables (e.g. poor mental health and social exclusion). Where there are testable hypotheses – which are predictions such as that higher levels of mental ill health are likely to be linked to higher levels of social exclusion – statistical tests can be used to establish relationships in these data, either through judging the strength of a difference or a correlation.

Qualitative research tends to emphasise words as data, such as the words of participants in interviews or written data from documents. Rather than testing hypotheses, qualitative research seeks to explain the meaning of social phenomena through exploring the ways in which individuals understand their social worlds. More recently, data in visual forms such as photographs or films have been an increasingly popular subject of study.

Epistemology: quantitative versus qualitative research

Terms such as 'epistemology' can seem very technical and a little daunting at first, but it is worth persevering as they are often not as complicated as they initially seem. Epistemology addresses the question of what constitutes valid knowledge, and it is helpful for understanding the different approaches to research that you will come across. A key division in research is between quantitative and qualitative research and each has its own epistemological approach. In its simplest formulation, quantitative research asks, 'what is going on here?' or 'which option is better than the other?' Qualitative research, on the other hand, asks 'what is the meaning of what is happening?' For example, a quantitative study may measure the rates for mental ill health and social exclusion for a sample of mental health service users and find that there is a link (i.e. people with higher rates of mental ill health are likely to experience higher rates of social exclusion). A qualitative study would explore the meaning of what is happening, for example whether people with mental health problems are experiencing stigma and prejudice, whether participants are isolating themselves as a means of coping with distressing symptoms or some other explanation. Both approaches can provide useful insights into a particular research topic and there is a growing recognition of the strengths of mixed methodologies (Cresswell, 2021). Actually, neither approach is 'better' than the other; it is simply deciding which is more appropriate for the research question, and the question should come before the choice of methodology because the type of question asked determines how it will be investigated. When planning a research project or developing a proposal for a module or in a clinical setting, deciding on your research question leads you to choose a research approach which is best suited to answering it. Qualitative and quantitative research approaches are considered in more detail later in the book.

Quantitative research

Quantitative research tends to follow a traditional scientific model, which emphasises 'objectivity' by seeking to remove the values and attitudes of the researcher from the study. There is an emphasis on studying causal relationships and formulating fixed rules for the process of inquiry. Sampling issues are particularly important because of the emphasis on being able to create statistical generalisations that are applicable to the wider population.

Quantitative research and positivism

Quantitative research has been influenced by *positivism* as an approach to knowledge. Every approach to research has underlying assumptions about the nature of knowledge and the social world, which is referred to as its *epistemological position*. Positivism as an epistemological position traces its intellectual heritage back to Auguste Comte and argues that the traditional scientific method applied in the natural sciences is appropriate to the study of society. From a positivist stance, the researcher is seen as an objective observer whose role is to infer laws that explain relationships between observed phenomena (Giddens and Sutton, 2021).

Gray (2017) identifies three major claims of positivism:

1. Reality is viewed as consisting only of what can be experienced through the senses. Consequently, phenomena that cannot directly be sensed (e.g. people's intentions, wishes and fears) are not suitable as a subject for scientific inquiry.

2. Inquiry should be based upon scientific observations rather than philosophical speculation, and therefore on empirical inquiry.

3. The natural and human sciences are similar as they share common logical and methodological principles. This includes the belief that facts can be distinguished from values.

Although positivism dominated the social sciences for much of the twentieth century, it has fallen from favour since the 1980s, as critics have challenged its core assumptions and its appropriateness for researching the complexities of our social world.

The challenges to positivism have led to a more sophisticated version of the traditional scientific approach known as realism, which is becoming increasingly influential. This is a broad range of approaches variously named as 'scientific realism', 'critical realism', 'subtle realism' and 'transcendental realism', each of which has a slightly different emphasis (Robson, 2016). An increasingly popular approach is critical realism (Bhaskar, 1978, 1979, 1990), which believes that there is an external reality but sees the concepts that we use to understand it as a provisional way of knowing rather than a direct reflection of reality. This approach also allows for theoretical content that is not amenable to direct observation, which would not be acceptable in positivism (Clark et al., 2021).

You are likely to come across the randomised controlled trial (RCT) in your literature reviews, as this is a particularly influential research approach in healthcare and nursing, involving what is known as an experimental design. We will discuss experimental designs and RCTs briefly below and then further in Chapter 6, but in essence they are ways of assessing the effectiveness of different 'treatments' to find out which one works best relative to others. They are increasingly popular and reported in nursing journals for all branches and specialities in nursing and are frequently described as the 'gold standard' in healthcare research.

Qualitative research

Qualitative research tends to use data in the form of words rather than numerical information. It seeks to explain social phenomena through understanding the ways in which individuals make sense of their social worlds and sees knowledge as historically and culturally situated. In qualitative research, there are no clearly defined rules about sample size, but generally smaller sample sizes are used and studied in more depth and detail. The primary focus is the importance of understanding individuals' own accounts of their perceptions, views and feelings and the meanings they attach to social phenomena.

Qualitative research and interpretivism

Qualitative research has been influenced by *interpretivism* as an epistemological position. Interpretivism is a broad term used to describe a range of approaches that challenge the traditional scientific approach of positivism. Interpretivism argues that the research methods of the natural sciences (from where positivism originated) are inappropriate to study social phenomena because they do not take into account the viewpoints of the social actors involved. For example, identifying the reasons for young people's unhealthy behaviour, such as drug taking or unprotected sex, requires the nurse researcher to understand the perspectives of those key social actors. The intellectual origins of interpretivism can be traced back to the nineteenth and early twentieth centuries as thinkers began to develop ways of researching, understanding and interpreting people's experiences of life (Clark et al., 2021).

Quantitative research is generally more valued by governmental bodies as it focuses more on 'what works' and is more easily generalisable. Medical research uses this approach extensively whereas nursing research has tended to favour qualitative approaches. More recently, there has been a trend towards combining these methodologies, so traditional distinctions have become blurred.

Qualitative research and reflexivity

Whereas quantitative research seeks to remove the researcher from the study through addressing issues of bias, qualitative researchers argue that this is neither possible nor necessarily desirable. We bring our background and identity to our research, but from a traditional perspective this is viewed as a problem (a source of bias) rather than a valuable component of the research (Maxwell, 2013). In qualitative research, this is developed through the concept of *reflexivity*, which acknowledges that we bring our own thoughts, values and beliefs as well as our ethnicity, race, class, gender, sexual orientation, occupation, family background and education to our research.

Reflexivity has been defined as the *practice of researchers being self-aware of their own beliefs, values and attitudes, and their personal effects on the setting they have studied, and self-critical about their research methods and how they have been applied* (Payne and Payne, 2004, page 191). Reflexivity can ensure high standards because it involves the researcher constantly reviewing the process of investigation. Huberman and Miles (2008) argue for the researcher documenting the research process. This has been referred to as an 'audit trail', which explains why decisions were made (Lincoln and Guba, 1985) and should be regarded as a resource rather than a defensive action (Payne and Payne, 2004).

Feminist research has a long tradition of promoting qualitative research as an appropriate strategy for studying social phenomena in context. Feminist research is not so much a specific research design or method, but an approach to research that is informed by a set of values. These values recognise the power differentials that exist within wider society and within academic discourses, which have favoured patriarchal models of research that emphasise objectivity and distance between the researcher and the researched. It emphasises reflexivity as part of the rejection of these models, and as a resource for a radical paradigm shift (Payne and Payne, 2004). Feminist research tends to be antipositivist, although it includes quantitative as well as qualitative research methods. It places gender at the centre of social inquiry, investigating and representing the diversity of women's perspectives (Sarantakos, 2013).

Generic qualitative research

When undertaking research studies using the designs listed below under the heading 'Research designs from particular traditions', it is necessary to adhere to these designs quite scrupulously, or rigour can suffer. More recently, a trend among some qualitative researchers is for what has become known as 'generic qualitative research' (Caelli et al., 2003). This is an approach that uses methods of data collection from the qualitative tradition, without some of the other methodological assumptions that come with the traditional qualitative schools of thought.

So, in summary, qualitative research is an approach which seeks to understand people's experiences in particular situations. This is useful in nursing because it can give us insight into the issues involved in, for example, living with illnesses, or being a patient or client and using services, or being marginalised or disadvantaged in some way. With an enhanced understanding of these areas, nurses can begin to think through how they can alter their care and tailor their services more effectively to meet the needs of their patients and clients. Such studies are usually quite small-scale and based in a local context, so we cannot automatically assume that the findings relate exactly to our own care settings, but qualitative work is often used where little is known about particular issues and it is a start (at least) to know things from small, local studies.

For those undertaking modules and planning projects, a research question seeking to understand or interpret people's experiences will lead to the use of a qualitative approach. This may be useful when little is known in an area of your own interest in practice, or as an attempt to evaluate issues in your own care setting or relating to your own service delivery. We look at qualitative designs in more detail in Section 3.

Activity 1.2   Reflection

Take a sheet of blank paper and try to answer the following questions based upon the material above:

1. What is meant by the terms 'epistemology' and 'epistemological stance'?
2. What are the differences between quantitative and qualitative research?

As this is a personal reflective activity using material from the chapter, there is no outline answer at the end of the chapter.

Research designs from particular traditions

When planning your project or undertaking a literature review, you will need to be able to identify and understand a range of research designs from different traditions. What follows is a brief introduction to these, which will help you gain an overview before starting your project. This is not exhaustive, neither is it intended as a menu from which you must choose. The aim is to illustrate the rich diversity in approaches to research design and the values that underpin them. The approaches are discussed in alphabetical order to challenge the idea that some designs are 'better' than others. To reiterate, the 'best' research design is the one that allows you to answer your research question.

We have suggested further reading for each of the designs covered below at the end of the chapter.

Action research and participatory action research

Action research challenges the traditional conception of the researcher as separate from the real world seeking theoretical knowledge that makes little difference in practice. It is associated with smaller-scale research projects that seek to address real-world problems, particularly among practitioners who want to improve practice, with a more equal and collaborative relationship between researchers and participants occurring as a feature of the study design. Rather than merely studying the social world, action research seeks to change it in practical ways. Another feature of action research is a view of the research process as being cyclical, in the sense that findings are fed back directly into practice in an ongoing process (Denscombe, 2014).

Action research traces its intellectual history to the work of Kurt Lewin, a social psychologist working in poor communities in post-Second World War America. Action research is not a specific research method. It is more an approach to research that stresses the importance of links with real-world problems and a belief that research should serve practical ends. It is compatible with a wide range of research methods, ranging from experimental to phenomenological designs.

Participatory action research (PAR) is a form of action research that is committed to the involvement of those who are most affected (Alston and Bowles, 2012). It challenges the traditional power imbalance between the researcher as 'expert' and research participant as 'passive subject' and is highly compatible with antidiscriminatory and antioppressive practice, as the focus is to change participants' situations for the better under their direction.

There are also a number of similar approaches, such as 'appreciative inquiry' and 'cooperative inquiry'. These share a commitment to promoting the empowerment of participants, but each has a different emphasis (Ludema et al., 2013).

Koch et al. (2008) illustrate how a PAR study can be used to give a voice to those who are usually marginalised, as well as to illuminate practice issues and day-to-day changes. They studied how women with multiple sclerosis (MS) and urinary incontinence perceive the daily challenges they encounter. Four female MS sufferers, the researcher and two continence nurse advisers (CNAs) met on five occasions and the group interactions were recorded and transcribed. As well as finding four themes in the interactions (maintaining control; seeking understanding; avoiding shame; and good and bad days), the women and the CNAs were able to discuss living with MS and incontinence from their differing perspectives. The CNAs learnt much about the women's experience and have changed their daily practice as a result.

These are fascinating and increasingly influential forms of research, but if you are choosing this for a method in your project plan, be aware that their innovative nature can make them problematic if they are not fully understood by students and supervisors, or if timescales are limited by the need to adhere to strict deadlines. Genuine participatory research requires considerable time to develop because the project's development is steered in the directions in which participants want to take it. This makes it difficult to predict at the outset where it will end up and how long it will take to achieve change; this uncertainty can involve ethical issues too (Williamson and Prosser, 2002).

Case studies

A *case study* is a detailed inquiry into a single example of a phenomenon, whether it is an organisation, individual, event, process, location or period of time (David, 2006). Rather than a research method, it is more a focus of study in which a variety of research methods can be used. These can range from experimental methods within a quantitative approach through to ethnography using observation and interviews within a qualitative approach. In practice, however, most case studies tend to adopt a qualitative approach (Payne and Payne, 2004) and are relatively descriptive.

Yin (2018) argues that case study research has traditionally been regarded as a 'weak sibling' compared to other research designs, such as experimental studies. This has changed in recent years as qualitative research has become more accepted within health and social sciences. A traditional criticism of case studies is whether findings can be generalised. For example, the statistical generalisations produced by large-scale statistical analysis would not be possible from a case study; this would be inappropriate because the case is studied in its own right rather than as an example of a particular class (Payne and Payne, 2004).

Yin (2018) identifies three types of case study. The *critical case* is chosen because it has features that challenge an existing theory or hypothesis. The *unique case* is chosen because its distinctiveness is its merit, although it may provide ways of understanding more usual cases. The *revelatory case* is chosen because it can provide new insights and ideas.

Courtenay et al. (2009) conducted a case study to explore issues in consultations between nurse prescribers and dermatology patients, as they wanted to illustrate the unique contribution of nurses to patient care. Ten practice settings were evaluated using a mixed-methods approach, including questionnaires, interviews and videoed observations of consultations. The researchers found that nurses believed their holistic approach to assessment and prescribing improved prescribing decisions, while patients valued nurses' skills in listening and in explaining treatments.

If you were choosing a case study approach you would need to be clear that you were investigating some aspect of local practice or patients' experiences, and that your research and findings would be highly context-specific and not necessarily relevant elsewhere. This does not mean that you should not conduct this type of research: it may be very useful and desirable that local service delivery or patients' experiences are evaluated and the findings shared more widely. These comments also apply to the discussion of evaluation research, below.

Clinical data mining

Clinical data mining (CDM) is a practice-based research strategy for systemically collecting and analysing available agency data such as medical, nursing, allied health and other hospital records (Epstein, 2009). CDM offers a promising and practical research approach for academics but is particularly attractive to research-minded practitioners and postgraduate degree students. For example, it can be used by practitioners to evaluate their own interventions and reflect upon their own practice. It is generally used retrospectively to analyse existing data but could be combined with original data collection. Likewise, it can provide data for master's and PhD degree studies on topics difficult to study via original data collection.

Epstein (2009) describes three basic types of CDM studies. The first type directly converts existing quantitative data to a quantitative database for statistical analysis. The second type converts data that were originally in narrative form (e.g. nursing notes) from qualitative form to a quantitative database for statistical analysis. The third type is purely qualitative data, where narrative data receive a qualitative analysis.

Case study 1.1: Data use in transplant suitability assessment

Patients with life-threatening liver disease go through a two-stage process at the Mount Sinai Medical Center in New York City to determine their eligibility for transplants. After they are determined as medically appropriate for transplant, patients then have a second assessment to determine their suitability for a transplant on psychosocial grounds. Since the shortage of donor organs means that only about half of requests can be accepted, the psychosocial assessment is crucial for patients. Staff team members and a research consultant extracted quantitative data about psychosocial risk factors and outcomes from around 500 former patients in order to complete the largest retrospective study of patient psychosocial risk factors and liver transplant mortality ever completed in the transplant literature (Epstein et al., 1997).

CDM has a number of strengths. First, it is practitioner-friendly, and it explicitly promotes practitioners as researchers. Second, it is less resource-intensive than most other forms of research. Since the data are already available, the costly and time-consuming process of data collection is avoided, although data will usually need work to convert them into a suitable format. Third, it makes use of valuable data that already exist but which are rarely used for research purposes. Since the amount of data that is collected for research purposes is only a tiny fraction of the amount of data routinely collected for clinical purposes, the potential for knowledge creation is considerable. Finally, CDM is unobtrusive and more ethically sound than most other data-gathering approaches. It does not involve the patient risks or burdens involved in data collection (e.g. interviewing patients, relatives or staff about sensitive topics), nor does it involve the ethical risks involved in experimental or quasi-experimental studies (see below for more detailed discussion). The main limitation of CDM is that any research method that relies on clinical records is only as good as the available data sources themselves. Consequently, missing data, reliability questions and absent variables must be anticipated. However, once recognised, these issues can be minimised with proper safeguards.

Evaluation research

Evaluation research has become popular within healthcare as part of the drive for increased accountability of public services and the evidence-based practice agenda. Indeed, it is usually valued highly by practitioners, particularly when deciding between different interventions, allocating scarce resources or demonstrating that in-service innovations are effective.

To evaluate something is to assess its merits or worth. By definition, it cannot be value-neutral because there must be aims and standards against which something is judged. In real life, evaluation is also rarely value-neutral in the sense that it can be used for organisational purposes. For example, evaluations can be used to justify closing a service or to promote the wider organisation.

Evaluation research requires you to develop specific criteria, which can be an interesting and fraught process as different stakeholders can have different perspectives. Senior management may be interested in cost-effectiveness, adherence to national standards and National Institute for Health and Care Excellence (NICE) guidelines, while service users may be more interested in how responsive the service is to their needs. There are obvious similarities with action research. However, one common difference is the role of the researcher. While the researcher in action research is often in a practitioner role, this is less acceptable within evaluation research because it would be viewed as compromising objectivity.

Another related criticism of evaluation is that it is atheoretical in its approach; that is, it does not use wider theory drawn from the social sciences to inform its design. In many contexts, this is not problematic, and studies do not need to demonstrate engagement with the wider academic literature in order to be effective and useful, provided that methods of data collection and analysis are rigorous. A final note of caution is that evaluation research can be politically sensitive, which can pose challenges for access and for researchers' relationships with service users and staff.

Service evaluations may utilise existing data and are similar in that respect to audit, or they may collect new data for a specific purpose. For example, Williamson et al. (2007) discuss a patient satisfaction survey of a nurse-led clinic for cancer care follow-up. Data were collected using a questionnaire, which evaluated the initial months of the clinic's existence. It was a new service and the nurse specialist and medical consultant wanted to understand the issues for patients and gain some perspective concerning what worked well, what might need to be altered, and what patients thought of the new service compared to the old medical-led arrangements. Overall, patients were satisfied with many aspects of the new service. While this service evaluation is highly context-specific, it illustrates how service redesign can take place as a result of national policy and clinical guidance, which had driven the changes. So, while Williamson et al.'s (2007) study evaluated satisfaction with the new service, they also generated some more widely applicable knowledge of relevance to similar services elsewhere or for the service user group as a whole.

Service evaluation is an important and growing area of healthcare research. Choosing a service evaluation as a project or for a proposal will allow you to gain skills in this area, which may come in useful at a later stage in your career when you have more responsibility for service delivery. It may suit you that you will not need to adopt a theoretical position (such as grounded theory or phenomenology) if the aim of your research is to produce useable findings for understanding and improving patient care.

Experimental and quasi-experimental designs

These designs are similar to a traditional scientific approach and are most often used to evaluate interventions and test theories (known as *hypotheses*). It is sometimes stated that an experimental design is the most rigorous form of research, which is somewhat misleading as all forms of research can possess rigour. It is more accurate to say that this is the approach that places most emphasis on removing possible sources of bias, which is achieved through introducing a degree of randomisation at different stages of the process, and by 'blinding' participants and staff to which intervention is being offered (known as 'double-blinding') where possible.

The classic experimental design is the RCT, mentioned earlier in the chapter, in which participants are randomly assigned to one of two groups: an experimental and a control group. The experimental group receives the intervention, whereas the control group does not, and the effects are then measured in each group. Having a control group receiving no intervention raises ethical issues, because it requires one group to not receive a potentially beneficial intervention. This is less ethically problematic when there is little evidence to date that the intervention is effective but becomes more so as there is evidence that participants would be likely to benefit, and so a new treatment could be compared to an existing one. So, for example, if researchers wanted to answer the question, 'What is the best treatment for high blood pressure?' they would investigate this by giving one medication to one group of patients and comparing the outcomes with another drug given to another group of similar patients. Statistical tests would be used to establish the importance of these outcomes and whether or not they could be generalised to a wider population from the sample in which they were observed.

RCTs form one end of a spectrum of experimental and quasi-experimental approaches that can be used. We discuss the distinctions between experimental and quasi-experimental designs more fully in Section 3: briefly, a full experimental design would contain more rigorous features than a quasi-experimental design, such as double-blinding (where neither researcher nor patients would know which new treatment was given to avoid any subliminal biases being introduced), or a control group who were receiving no treatment or an existing one for the purposes of comparison. A common quasi-experimental design is a pre- and post-test design, in which one group of participants experiences an intervention and key variables are measured before and after the intervention to establish whether there has been a change. Quasi-experiments also fre-quently do not undertake randomisation.

For example, Chiang and Sun (2009) investigated whether introducing a walking programme for Chinese Americans would reduce their hypertension (high blood pres-sure) rates, with one group experiencing the programme, and another experiencing a culturally modified programme (aimed at being attractive to them as older Chinese Americans). There were no significant effects upon participant blood pressure or walking endurance as a result of both programmes, and the study indicated that the walking protocol is appropriate to use without additional cultural modification.

This study illustrates how a quasi-experimental design might be useful in investigat-ing variables which cannot rigorously be controlled or blinded: it was not possible to blind researchers and participants to allocated groups as patients were receiving dif-ferent input from researchers and behaving differently as a result. This was obvious to the researchers, meaning that the full experimental control associated with a true experimental design is not present in this study. If you are thinking about constructing an experimental design, it is worth noting that the full features (which we discuss in Section 3) do not need to be present, and although quasi-experimental designs are not as robust as fully experimental ones, they can be used successfully.

Narrative approaches

Narrative approaches are interested in the storied nature of human conduct, in which we respond to experiences by constructing stories and listening to the stories of others and there has been increasing interest in narrative approaches across the social sciences (Andrews et al., 2013).

Narratives have traditionally been viewed as discourses with a clear sequential order that connects events in a meaningful way for a definite audience and thus offer insights about the world. However, such definitions are in dispute and the process of analysis does not offer the tightly prescribed procedures prevalent in approaches such as grounded theory (Riessman, 2007; Andrews et al., 2013).

Elliott (2005, page 6) identifies the following common themes in narrative research:

- an interest in people's lived experiences and an appreciation of the temporal nature of that experience;
- a desire to empower research participants and allow them to contribute to determining the most salient themes in the area of research;
- an interest in process and change over time;
- an interest in the self and representations of the self;
- an awareness that the researcher him- or herself is also a narrator.

Narrative research is often interested in issues of identity as stories play a central role in the formation of identity (Crossley, 2007, page 135). Indeed, Mair asserts that:

> *Stories are the womb of personhood. Stories make and break us. Stories sustain us in times of trouble and encourage us towards ends that we would not otherwise envision.*

> (Mair, 1989, page 2)

The history of narrative approaches to research can be traced back to two different academic traditions (Andrews et al., 2013). The first is the post-Second World War rise of humanistic approaches within psychology and sociology as a reaction against positivism. The second is the influence within the humanities of a range of developments from Russian structuralist, French poststructuralist, postmodern, psychoanalytic and deconstructionist approaches to narrative (Andrews et al., 2013).

There is a range of approaches to narrative research and a commonly made distinction is between event-centred and experience-centred approaches. Event-centred approaches focus upon the spoken recounting of particular past events that happened to the narrator (Andrews et al., 2013), and are influenced by the work of Labov (Labov and Waletsky, 1967). Experience-centred approaches have a broader focus and explore stories that may be about general or imagined phenomena, things that happened to the narrator or distant matters that they have only heard about and can include writing and visual materials as well as speech (Andrews et al., 2013).

The interest in people's lived experiences and in questions of identity mean that narrative research is particularly appropriate for understanding the experiences of trauma and researching sensitive issues (Crossley, 2000, 2007). Examples of narrative research include a study of the use of therapeutic letters in family therapy (Curtis et al., 2002) and a study of families affected by the government's Troubled Families initiative (Wills et al., 2017).

If you were going to choose a narrative approach for your own study or proposal, this could be a good way of giving a voice to people who are not usually heard and to engage in a long dialogue with many people, particularly if the potential of electronic communications, such as e-mail, is utilised sensitively and effectively to interact with participants (Kralik et al., 2006).

A research attitude

Whichever research approach and design are chosen, it is important for you as a researcher to develop a 'research attitude'. This is about being rigorous in your thinking and willing to challenge yourself and others in a responsible way. This has been expressed by Robson (2016) as follows:

- Being systematic: giving serious thought to what is being done and how and why it is being done. This involves considering alternatives and making an argument for the choices made.
- Being sceptical: subjecting ideas to scrutiny and possible disconfirmation. This involves researchers asking themselves what evidence exists for the points they are making and considering alternative explanations.
- Being ethical: working within acceptable parameters. This involves following ethical frameworks, particularly those of the Health Research Authority and the NHS Trust research governance processes, as well as thinking about how their research might affect others (Robson, 2016), the potential clinical significance of their work and the need to comply with the requirements of professional bodies such as the NMC (Williamson, 2001).

Chapter summary

This chapter has asked you to reflect upon your initial thoughts about engaging in research. You have been introduced to key terms in research, and the distinction between quantitative and qualitative approaches to research was discussed. You have been asked to consider a range of research designs from particular traditions to illustrate the wide diversity of approaches.

In the next chapter we will look at how to undertake a literature review and appraise and use research to inform practice.

Further reading

General

Clark, T, Foster, L, Bryman, A and Sloan, L (2021) *Bryman's Social Research Methods* (6th edition). Oxford: Oxford University Press.

An excellent, all-round textbook that covers all aspects of the research process, including chapters on different methods (such as experimental and non-experimental methods).

Ellis, P (2023) *Evidence-Based Practice in Nursing* (5th edition). London: Sage/Learning Matters.

A clear and simple book which helps develop skills in the identification, appraisal and application of evidence for nursing practice.

Kvale, S and Brinkmann, S (2014) *InterViews: Learning the Craft of Qualitative Research Interviewing* (2nd edition). London: Sage.

Second edition of a classic text, mainly considering the qualitative approach, which provides an interesting and detailed account of the differences between positivist and interpretative approaches.

Parahoo, K (2014) *Nursing Research: Principles, Process and Issues* (3rd edition). Basingstoke: Palgrave Macmillan.

Comprehensive research methods' text.

Action research and participatory action research

Coghlan, D and Brannick, T (2019) *Doing Action Research in Your Own Organisation* (5th edition). London: Sage.

A very good text, dealing succinctly with key issues, including methodology and implementation.

Reason, P and Bradbury, H (eds) (2013) *Handbook of Action Research* (2nd edition). London: Sage.

A useful collection of chapters by key figures in action research.

Williamson, GR, Bellman, L and Webster, J (2012) *Action Research in Nursing and Healthcare.* London: Sage.

This is an excellent resource for nurses and other healthcare professionals seeking to understand and use action research in their clinical practice.

Case studies

Yin, R (2018) *Case Study Research: Design and Methods* (6th edition). London: Sage.

The classic text on case study design.

Clinical data mining

Epstein, I (2010) *Clinical Data-Mining: Integrating Practice and Research.* New York: Oxford University Press.

An excellent and interesting account of a new approach to documentary analysis. An insightful and entertaining read.

Evaluation research

Hall, I and Hall, D (2004) *Evaluation and Social Research: Introducing Small-Scale Practice.* Basingstoke: Palgrave Macmillan.

A useful guide that presents practical advice and real-life examples.

Pawson, R and Tilley, N (1997) *Realistic Evaluation.* London: Sage.

A classic and provocative text from the realist tradition.

Experimental and quasi-experimental designs

Clark, T, Foster, L, Bryman, A and Sloan, L (2021) *Bryman's Social Research Methods* (6th edition). Oxford: Oxford University Press.

An excellent resource for students using social science research methods.

Parahoo, K (2014) *Experiments, in Nursing Research: Principles, Process and Issues* (3rd edition). Basingstoke: Palgrave Macmillan.

One of the seminal texts on research methods for nurses.

Narrative approaches

Andrews, M, Squire, C and Tamboukou, M (eds) (2013) *Doing Narrative Research* (2nd edition). London: Sage.

An excellent introduction to both the theoretical and practical dimensions of narrative research.

Riessman, C (2007) *Narrative Methods for the Human Sciences.* London: Sage.

An updated version of the classic 1993 text.

Useful websites

Organisations conducting and using research

www.jrf.org.uk

The Joseph Rowntree Foundation. Independent research foundation with useful publications on many subjects, including health and healthcare, poverty and social exclusion.

www.kingsfund.org.uk

The King's Fund. An independent charity seeking to improve healthcare. See their publications.

www.nice.org.uk

The National Institute for Health and Care Excellence. Provides clinical guidance on healthcare issues.

www.nihr.ac.uk

The National Institute for Health Research. Commissions and funds NHS and social care research and develops research evidence to support decision making by professionals.

www.rcn.org.uk/professional-development/research-and-innovation

The Royal College of Nursing Research and Development Co-ordinating Centre. Facilitates rather than conducts research but aims to increase the capacity of nurses working in research.

www.wellcome.ac.uk

The Wellcome Trust. A charity that funds medical and humanities research.

Research methods sources

https://researchmethodscommunity.sagepub.com

Sage Research Methods Community. Research methods community resources and blog produced by Sage Publishing.

Section 2

Planning and preparing for your final-year project

Chapter 2 Planning and undertaking a literature review

Chapter aims

After reading this chapter, you should be able to:

- understand what a literature review is;
- feel confident about undertaking a literature search;
- be able to source high-quality material in your topic area.

Introduction

You will have had some thoughts about your research topic and be starting to formulate your research question. The next stage is to undertake a literature review in order to establish what is already known about your research topic. This chapter aims to guide you through the process, using case studies and activities to illustrate the different stages. This is a distinct process from conducting a systematic review and meta-analysis, which is a literature review undertaken using a strict, explicit, and transparent set of formal protocols that seek to minimise the chances of systematic bias and error (Gough et al., 2017). We devote Chapter 8 to an introduction to systematic reviews and meta-analyses.

It is important to see your literature review as an ongoing process that would start in the early stages of planning your proposal, and would continue throughout the life of your project, if you were actually undertaking one. This would not be just about updating your literature review as new material becomes available: if you were undertaking data collection, these data would be likely to suggest new ways of looking at your research topic. Consequently, developing your literature review would be a continual process, in which you re-engaged with the literature as your project developed.

This chapter will begin by defining what is meant by a literature review and exploring its roles and functions. The process of undertaking a *literature search* will be reviewed, focusing on the challenge of finding high-quality material in your topic area. Chapter 10 looks at how a literature review can be written up.

The procedures for undertaking a literature search and making effective notes will be examined. You will be asked to consider what it means to analyse critically the literature that you find, and clear guidelines will be discussed. The process of writing up your literature review will be considered and some of the problems frequently encountered by students will be examined.

What is a literature review?

A literature review is a comprehensive summary and critical appraisal of the literature that is relevant to your research topic. It presents the reader with what is already known in this field and identifies traditional and current controversies as well as weaknesses and gaps in the field.

The terms *literature search* and *literature review* are sometimes treated as if they were synonymous, but a literature search refers to a systematic process of identifying material that is appropriate whereas a literature review refers to a critical evaluation of that material.

In a dissertation involving data collection, you will discuss what you found in the body of literature at two stages. First, you will present it in your literature review to demonstrate your understanding of what has already been written in your field. This will be used to inform your study design. You then revisit it after your findings to discuss any similarities and differences between what you found and what previous researchers have found. In a proposal, you will only use the literature to create an introductory argument or give background to the study, which will also inform the study design.

Hart (2018) identifies two key areas when you begin a research project or write a proposal: the literature relevant to your research topic and the literature on research *methodology* (i.e. how to plan and conduct research). This is an important distinction because you are likely to have only searched for the former during your previous academic study. Reading this book is an excellent start to developing your knowledge of the latter and each chapter contains recommended texts for further reading.

There are many reasons for undertaking a literature review. It is an essential part of your project planning and would form a necessary part of any project you might actually undertake. A systematic review and meta-analysis might also be acceptable for master's qualification instead of an empirical research project (i.e. where you collect your own data), and might form part of a dissertation or extended study project in third-year undergraduate nursing programmes. It enables you to gain an understanding of what has already been written about your topic, including reviewing which research designs have been used and the key issues that have been identified. Consequently, it is an essential part of developing expertise in your field, both in the topic area and in research methodology, and will inform your project plan.

Conducting your literature search

A literature search is the first stage in your literature review and is an organised investigation for material relevant to your topic across a range of sources. In your previous studies, you may have concentrated on using textbooks to inform your coursework. The purpose of textbooks is to provide students with an overview of what is generally agreed in a particular field. Although textbooks may report the results of research studies, they may not be sufficiently current or detailed for the purposes of your literature review. You need to expand the range of literature that you utilise, and this should include reading the original research studies themselves to be able to appraise them critically.

Types of literature

The main types of literature that will be relevant are described below.

Journal articles in printed and electronic form

These are generally regarded as being of the highest quality because most journals are peer-reviewed. This means that articles submitted to the journals will be anonymised and sent out to reviewers with expertise in the field. These reviewers will evaluate the potential article and will submit detailed feedback that the author must address before it is of a publishable standard. This does not guarantee that everything in an article is correct, but it is relatively stringent. While articles from non-refereed journals may be of a similar standard, they have not been through this process. Journals will state that they are peer-reviewed if this is the case and many search engines allow you to search for refereed journals only.

Books in printed and electronic form

There are good-quality control mechanisms built into book publishing, but they are not regarded as being as stringent as for peer-reviewed journals. You may be used to reading textbooks that provide you with a good overview of an area, but the research studies that they describe are likely to be classic studies rather than the most recent material.

Official and legal publications

These include legislation, policy and discussion documents as well as research studies and summaries of research findings in specific subject areas, such as hospital discharge or child protection. As well as governmental bodies, this includes material from other public organisations such as the Nuffield Foundation, the Joseph Rowntree Foundation, or the National Society for the Prevention of Cruelty to Children (NSPCC).

Systematic reviews, meta-analyses and clinical guidelines

Systematic reviews and *meta-analyses* are exceptionally influential in medical, nursing and healthcare research as they inform decision making and treatment options on a daily basis and provide an evidence base for the national recommendations for standards of treatment and care produced by NICE and other bodies, such as the Scottish Intercollegiate Guidelines Network (SIGN). The most important and influential body funding systematic reviews and meta-analyses is the Cochrane Collaboration, and there is a Cochrane Nursing Care organisation. The Joanna Briggs Institute is also a good resource for nurses. The purpose of systematic reviews of the literature is to find all relevant evidence on a pre-defined question by employing a rigorous search process that is free from author bias, to assess the rigour of the studies and to combine their results into a meaningful conclusion that can also serve as a guide to clinical practice and the need for further research.

Clinical guidelines can be extremely authoritative if published by influential bodies such as NICE and SIGN and have gone through extensive processes of literature search and review before conclusions relating to effectiveness and cost-effectiveness of new treatments are given. Many NHS Trusts develop their own guidelines, which go through clinical governance approval, but that does not necessarily mean that they are completely authoritative.

Grey literature

This is material that is not published through traditional commercial sources but is available through specialised sources (e.g. research reports from local public or voluntary organisations). It is often unclear what quality control systems have been used, but they may contain some very useful and relevant information. University libraries will have copies of doctoral and master's theses submitted at their institutions, and conference abstracts may be useful in identifying 'cutting-edge' work. Whether to include them in your literature review depends upon what other material you have found and whether your university expects you to include it. If you have found similar material from more conventional sources, you may not need to include them. But such material can be very valuable as long as you recognise the relative authority and its strengths and weaknesses.

How do I start my literature search?

The focal point of your literature search will be a systematic examination of a number of electronic bibliographic databases, which will enable you to search effectively across a large number of journals. These are available through your university library and are often available to access remotely through your home computer.

Most databases have 'basic' and 'advanced' search engines, so try using the latter for more specific and detailed searches and combine your key words to find more relevant results. When you search using an electronic database, you will be provided with an abstract that summarises the study. If your university has a subscription to that journal, you will also be able to get access to the full-text version. The content of most electronic databases consists of journal articles, but some may include references to other material, such as books, reports and websites. Since no bibliographic database contains every journal available, you will need to search a number of databases to ensure that you identify all of the material available. Google Scholar is also useful and recommended, although it is likely to throw up thousands of hits, of which only a few will be relevant. You should also search the Cochrane Collaboration website and the NHS Evidence website.

It is tempting to start searching immediately, but you should first put together a search profile. This will direct your search and should consist of the following:

- Your research question: this guides every aspect of your project. For example, 'What are the reasons for delays in hospital discharge for older people?' Make sure you express the research question as a full sentence with a question mark at the end.
- Key words: these are the main terms that relate to your research question, which you will use as search terms. They should include alternative terms that may be used in the literature; for example, using 'older people' but also alternative (and often out-of-date) terms such as 'elderly' or 'geriatric'.
- Parameters: these are any restrictions that will narrow down your search, such as a particular time period or country of research or factors related to the population studied (e.g. age, gender and ethnicity); for example, deciding that you want literature on hospital discharge delay from the UK and relating to older people rather than other age groups.
- PICO: The mnemonic PICO (Sackett et al., 1997) is a useful means of structuring a search. PICO stands for:
  - **P**opulation (or illness or condition);
  - **I**ntervention (treatment or service);
  - **C**ontrol (or comparison);
  - **O**utcome.
- Using PICO to write down for yourself exactly what you are searching for allows you to structure your search very clearly and make sure you do not go off track. You will always have a population (or illness or condition) in your search; you may not always have an intervention in the sense of a treatment option, but this could also relate to service delivery; you may not have a control (comparison) unless experimental designs are involved, and the outcomes may not be clearly articulated

at the search stage. Even so, PICO can help plan your literature search. Another useful mnemonic is SPIDER (Cooke et al., 2012). This stands for:

o **S**ample;

o **P**henomenon of **I**nterest;

o **D**esign;

o **E**valuation;

o **R**esearch type.

Case study 2.1: Developing key words

Jane decided that the research question that she is most interested in discovering literature on is identifying best practice in falls' prevention for elderly people living in residential homes. For her literature search, her first task is to develop a list of key words that she is going to use.

Activity 2.1   Critical thinking

What will Jane include in her search profile? What will she include in her research question, key words and parameters? What will she include in her PICO assessment?

There is a brief summary of answers at the end of the chapter.

It can be confusing and frustrating at first to use some electronic search engines because they use *Boolean operators*. This sounds technical, but it is a relatively simple system to enable you to narrow your search and find the most relevant resources. These are built into the advanced search functions, and it is worth understanding how they work. Although each database uses them in slightly different ways, the general principles apply.

The three most commonly used Boolean operators are 'AND', 'OR' and 'NOT'. If you insert the word 'AND' between search terms (e.g. 'elderly' AND 'falls') you will narrow your search to texts that contain both terms. If you insert the term OR between search terms, you will broaden your search to include texts that contain either term. These can usefully be combined; for example, 'elderly AND falls OR residential homes' will identify resources that discuss the elderly in the context of either falls or residential home settings. If you insert the term 'NOT' this will exclude any resources containing the second search term. This is useful when it has more than one meaning and you wish to restrict it. For example, if your search term is 'counselling' and you want to exclude careers' counselling, you would use 'counselling NOT careers counselling'. Another useful function is the truncation symbol (* ! #), which lets you type in the first part of a word and then the search engine will find alternative endings; for example, adolesc* will find adolescent, adolescents, adolescence, and so on.

It is important to be systematic about your searches to ensure that you have identified all the relevant literature. Having all of your material in one place means that you will not have to search through different notebooks or diaries to find a reference. This should include all the searches that you undertake, including the date, bibliographic database and search terms used. A popular format is an electronic word-processing document with dated entries that enable you to track the progress of your research and to search for specific words. If you prefer to work on physical copies, consider having a folder of A4 sheets that can be taken out and placed into a ring binder as you go along. Whichever format you choose, you should maintain regular electronic or photocopied back-ups to ensure that the material is not lost.

Make a record of when you undertake a search, including the key words you used and date. You will need to use more than one database because every database has a limited coverage. More importantly, make a reference list as you go along so that you avoid having to search for a reference at the last minute. There are a number of reference manager software packages, such as Mendeley, EndNote, ProCite and RefWorks; some are available as web versions as well as desktop applications, and these will allow you to search for references and store the results of your searches and, importantly, to get the citation style exactly correct. Becoming familiar with these packages is relatively easy, and you can drop the citations you want directly into a Word document as you are writing. The software will create the reference lists for you. Your university is likely to have adopted a 'house style' for referencing, as have academic journals, and a software package will create a central database of references that can be adapted into different citation systems, meaning that you could automatically adjust all the references to your university's correct style, or even a new style if necessary. Such software allows you to store your articles in PDF format ('portable document format': articles which look exactly as if you have printed them from a journal) and can automatically input details of the articles, though it is important to check these for accuracy.

An additional search method that can be productive (but far less systematic) is to review the references' section of material that you have already obtained. This can be particularly helpful when you have found an article that directly responds to your research question, because the references' section is likely to include relevant material. As you gather more articles and books, you may find the same texts being referred to. This usually indicates that these are central texts for your topic and should be included in your literature review. This form of searching can be quite fruitful, but rather haphazard and biased because the writers may not be familiar with all of the literature and may not have included material that they want to distance themselves from. Hence, it should be regarded as a supplement rather than a replacement for a full literature search using electronic databases. You can try this trick with authors' names, so you search for everything that a particular author has written, then try the same thing with all the co-authors on their papers. You can usually do this in the electronic databases you will be using by clicking on the relevant buttons. Although not systematic, it does give you a feel for who is publishing what in a particular field.

Effective reading and note taking

Having identified suitable material, it is important that you are able to use effective reading and note-taking skills to make the most of the time that you have. Rather than printing everything and working your way through a large pile of material, use active reading skills to identify which material is most relevant and take appropriate notes. As you should be able to get electronic full-text PDFs, often it is not necessary to print the articles you find on paper if you are comfortable reading them on screen.

A classic technique for achieving this is known as the SQ3R reading strategy, which comprises the following five stages:

1. Survey (or skim): conduct a preliminary scan of the material to get a general sense of what the material is about. This may simply consist of reading the abstract if it is a journal article. Does it look relevant? If not, discard at this stage.

2. Question: actively ask yourself what the article or chapter is about and what questions it might answer in order to decide whether the text is worth reading more carefully.

3. Read the text more carefully if it has passed the above tests. Read actively, questioning the author's arguments, and make appropriate notes.

4. Recall (or recite) the main points when you have finished reading, using your own words.

5. Review: test yourself to see what you can recall. If there are sections that you cannot remember, you may need to reread the material.

One of the most useful tips for saving time and reducing stress is to make sure that you keep a note of the full reference for the material that you are reading. While this may seem like a nuisance at the time, it will be preferable to hunting around for it at the last minute, long after you originally read it. It is particularly important to keep the reference list of your proposal or project report up to date as you go along (unless you are using a reference manager software package such as Mendeley or EndNote, which will help you).

When you are reading and taking notes, try to make links with other material that you have read. When you read your first article, it is difficult to have a framework to judge it against. When you have read a number of articles, you will have a greater understanding of the literature and will find it easier to evaluate a particular article or book.

Case study 2.2: Recording searches

Susan developed a system for recording her literature searches and the material that she found. Using her research journal she recorded every search. She also noted the numbers of search hits and how she reduced large numbers of hits to those of more relevance to her interests, as these details are frequently needed in assignments and proposals, so that it can be shown that a search is systematic and inclusive rather than biased in some way.

Susan read the abstract of every article in order to gain a sense of what it contained. She decided to use a traffic light system to organise the material into three groups (red, amber and green lights). For some articles, reading the abstract was enough for her to realise that the article was not relevant to her research and was discarded at that stage (red light). Other articles looked very promising and highly relevant to her research topic so were grouped together (green light). A third group were articles that were potentially relevant, depending upon how her research developed (amber light). She decided to devote most of her attention to the 'green light' group in order to develop a good knowledge of her specific research topic but to keep material from the 'amber light' group in case her research changed as it developed.

If, like Susan, you used a traffic light system, you could mark all the printed papers and keep them together in a folder, or you could simply keep the PDFs in separate folders in your computer's memory. However, we strongly recommend using computer software such as EndNote or Mendeley, as it will allow you to catalogue very efficiently and insert citations directly into the text and reference list.

What if I find too much or too little material?

In literature searching it is highly unusual to get exactly what you want, in the quantity that you want it, first time around. Usually you will need to repeat searches in different databases, refine your search terms and search again and again. As you start your literature search, you may find yourself confronted with either too much or too little material. It is more common to find that your literature search has identified too much material. The development of digital technology has seen a revolution in the information that is available for your research compared to almost 20 years ago. The disadvantage of this is that it is easy to become overwhelmed by the sheer volume of information that is available. If you have identified too much material, your search is too broad and needs to be narrowed down. This can be done in a number of ways. First, you could be more specific about your topic. Second, you can be more specific about your parameters (e.g. choosing a specific time period or restricting your search to UK materials).

If you have identified too little material, you need to think about your search terms. Whereas some areas really do have very little written about them, it is more likely that your search terms are not fine-tuned enough to pick them up. If you have identified a small amount of material, read it to find out the terminology that is used in your research field. Think of alternative terms and enlist the help of your supervisor and/ or fellow students in this task. If you still cannot identify any literature in your research field, it may be necessary to consider adjusting your research topic to ensure you have sufficient material to discuss in your literature review. If you genuinely cannot find anything on a subject area you will need to look at related subject areas for justification, rationale and methodological ideas concerning how you write your proposal.

Critically analysing the literature

In order to be worth including in your literature search, a text needs to be both relevant and of sufficient quality. Avoid the pitfall of reading material that is interesting, but not directly relevant to your research. This can take up a considerable amount of your time and the material is unlikely to feature in your final dissertation.

When you are evaluating a research study, there are a number of questions that you should ask yourself:

- Research design: does the study provide a clear rationale for the choice of research design? Research questions can usually be approached using a variety of research designs so a good study will provide a clear and robust rationale for its choices, including a discussion of why it did not use alternative designs.
- Data-collection methods: does the study provide a clear rationale for the choice of data-collection methods? For example, a study may have chosen interviews rather than questionnaires or focus groups. Is a coherent account given for this choice? Were known weaknesses addressed and did the data-collection methods work in practice?
- Sampling: how well do the sampling procedures match the research question? Sampling is particularly important in quantitative research because this limits the extent to which the findings can be generalised. Were known weaknesses addressed and did the sampling procedures work in practice?
- Data analysis: how robust is the data analysis? A good study will give a clear account of how the data were analysed, whether quantitative or qualitative. Does the data analysis follow the model described? If it is a quantitative study using statistical analysis, are the tests used appropriate? Please see the end of the chapter for recommended texts on quantitative data analysis and the Research Methods Knowledge Base website to provide a useful guide to appropriate statistical tests. If it is a qualitative study, does the analysis provide sufficient context for the material to be understandable? Does it account for the diversity of participants' views?
- Credibility of the findings: how credible are the findings? You need to consider whether the conclusions are supported by sufficient evidence and whether they have a consistent logic. It is important to be rigorous about this, because we tend to view findings that we agree with as more credible.

- Generalisability of the findings: to what extent can the findings be generalised to other settings? For quantitative studies, statistical generalisation is important and this is linked to sampling procedures. For qualitative research, generalisation is not viewed in the same way and the important issue is whether the concepts that are generated are meaningful in other settings. Is the study clear about the extent to which its findings can be generalised to other settings? If so, does this seem reasonable given the limitations of the study?
- Research ethics: how does the study address ethical issues? This should include ethical procedures followed and address issues such as informed consent, ethical data management and how potential risks were avoided. It can also include discussion of the values that underpin the study.

Not all of the literature you identify will be research studies. They may be opinion pieces in which the authors put forward a particular argument or viewpoint based upon their experience or on previous literature. However, many of the same criteria are relevant. Is the argument plausible? What evidence do the authors provide to substantiate their claims? Sometimes you may find an article that provides a literature review of your topic area. This may be useful for understanding the key issues and authors. However, do not assume that the authors are coming from an impartial perspective. They may have an allegiance to a particular point of view or position and, consequently, they may place less emphasis on, or even ignore, literature that does not support their stance.

A number of frameworks for critiquing literature of all kinds, including empirical research studies, clinical guidelines and systematic reviews and meta-analyses, are available. For example, the Critical Appraisal Skills Programme (CASP) and the Joanna Briggs Institute (JBI) organisation have developed tools to help with the process of critically appraising articles. Some useful websites are suggested at the end of this chapter.

Chapter summary

This chapter began by defining what is meant by a literature review and exploring its roles and functions. The process of undertaking a literature search was reviewed, focusing on the challenge of finding high-quality material in your topic area.

The procedures for undertaking a literature search and making effective notes were examined. You were asked to consider what it means to analyse critically the literature that you find and clear guidelines have been discussed.

Activity: Brief outline answer

Activity 2.1 Critical thinking (literature searches) (page 38)

Jane is already clear about her research question, namely, 'What is best practice in falls' prevention for elderly people living in residential homes?' For her, the key words 'falls' prevention' and 'residential homes' were both relevant and were combined in the search using the Boolean operator 'AND' as she knew that searching using only 'falls' prevention' would have produced too many results. She wanted to include literature from outside the UK but was aware that she would need to restrict it to material in English, as this was her only language. Her PICO was as follows:

- population: elderly people living in residential homes;
- intervention: falls' prevention strategies;
- control (comparison): no strategy;
- outcome: rate of falls.

Further reading

Literature reviews

Aveyard, H (2023) *Doing a Literature Review in Health and Social Care: A Practical Guide* (5th edition). Berkshire: Open University Press.

A useful and rigorous account of conducting a literature review.

Cullum, N, Ciliska, D, Haynes, B and Marks, S (2007) *Evidence-Based Nursing: An Introduction.* Oxford: Wiley-Blackwell.

A useful and interesting guide to understanding evidence-based practice in nursing.

Ellis, P (2023) *Evidence-Based Practice in Nursing* (5th edition). London: Sage/Learning Matters.

More detailed information about evidence-based practice in nursing.

Fink, A (2019) *Conducting Research Literature Reviews: From the Internet to Paper* (5th edition). London: Sage.

A useful guide which focuses on evaluating quantitative research and provides an outline of appropriate statistical tests when appraising research evidence.

Greenhalgh, T (2019) *How to Read a Paper* (6th edition). London: BMJ Publishing.

A book-length guide to appraising research papers from both quantitative and qualitative traditions.

Greenhalgh, T and Taylor, R (1997) How to read a paper: papers that go beyond numbers (qualitative research). *British Medical Journal,* 315: 740–3.

A classic article that provides a clear account of evaluating qualitative research studies.

Hart, C (2018) *Doing a Literature Review: Releasing the Social Science Research Imagination* (3rd edition). London: Sage.

A classic introduction to compiling your literature review that gives detailed guidance on structure and evaluating arguments.

Useful websites

www.casp-uk.net

CASP has developed the following tools to help with the process of critically appraising articles:

- systematic reviews;
- RCTs;
- qualitative research;

- economic evaluation studies;
- cohort studies;
- case-control studies;
- diagnostic test studies;
- clinical prediction rules.

CASP also has a useful glossary of terms at **https://casp-uk.net/glossary/**.

https://jbi.global

JBI is a global organisation promoting evidence-based decision making in healthcare. The website has critical appraisal tools to assess the trustworthiness, relevance and results of published papers.

www.prisma-statement.org

PRISMA (Preferred Reporting Items for Systematic Reviews and Meta-Analyses) provides an evidence-based minimum set of items for reporting in systematic reviews and meta-analyses.

The Research Methods Knowledge Base (https://conjointly.com/kb/)

The Research Methods Knowledge Base is a comprehensive web-based textbook that addresses all of the topics in a typical introductory undergraduate or graduate course in social research methods.

https://bl.iro.bl.uk/collections/ British Library search engine for searching for PhD theses.

Chapter 3 Planning your research proposal or dissertation

Chapter aims

After reading this chapter, you should be able to:

- plan the stages of your research project;
- choose your research area or topic, and develop your research question with the help of concept maps;
- draw up a timetable for carrying out your research, and a list of resource issues;
- understand the basic ethical principles governing research, and how to seek approval for your study.

Introduction

This chapter looks at how you go about planning your research proposal or dissertation. We take you through the key issues: planning the stages of the research process; choosing your research area/topic and developing your research question using concept maps; developing a research plan and timetable and considering resource issues; and addressing ethical approval and research governance issues.

Planning your research

Planning your research properly takes time but this is an essential step which will help you to construct a convincing argument about why the research is worth doing and how you will do it. It is important in your planning to allow yourself sufficient time to undertake your research and allow for possible delays. For example, common delays occur when trying to obtain ethical approvals, or if participants cancel and you have to rearrange appointments. Similarly, transcribing interviews or focus groups takes longer than people anticipate and data analysis even more so, so this all needs to be reflected in the planning and timetabling of activities. As a novice researcher it would be worthwhile keeping a research journal or logbook in which you could jot down ideas, notes of material you have read, conversations that you have had and to-do lists. Postgraduate students are likely to be asked to keep a portfolio-type research log, which will contain all this information and be used at supervision meetings with supervisors. You could record all of your thoughts as your proposal develops and include the texts that you identify and the results of your literature searches. It would be invaluable in promoting reflexivity, as it enables you to capture and examine your thoughts on the research process, the decisions that you have made and your role as researcher. This is a particularly important process in qualitative research and should be built into qualitative proposals. There are six stages in research (see Table 3.1), which we will now explore in detail.

Table 3.1   The six stages of research

Phase	Stage
Phase 1: Planning.	Stage 1: Choosing your research topic and formulating your research question.
	Stage 2: Choosing your research approach. This will be the main focus of this chapter and consists of the following stages:
	• deciding your research approach – qualitative and quantitative research;
	• deciding your research design, including research method and sampling;
	• ethical approval.
	Stage 3: Undertaking the literature review.
Phase 2: Data collection.	Stage 4: Collecting your data.
Phase 3: Data analysis and writing it up.	Stage 5: Analysing your data. Making sense of the data that you obtain will be discussed in Chapter 7.
	Stage 6: Writing up your research.

Choosing your research topic and formulating your research question

The initial stage of the research process is choosing a research topic and developing it into a specific research question. Do not be tempted to formulate complicated questions on the basis that they sound academic. If you read classic research studies, you will find that they have worked well because they have chosen simple, focused research questions.

Your first task is to identify a research topic and formulate your research questions. While the former is often quite easy, the latter can be quite challenging. This is because most students have one or more general area of interest but translating this into specific research questions usually involves reformulation.

When choosing your research topic, there are three main considerations:

1. *What are you interested in studying?* You may choose a subject to research for a range of reasons, such as personal or professional experience, an interest in the academic subject and an awareness of a gap in the literature. Choose a subject that you are genuinely interested in, otherwise it is difficult to maintain enthusiasm over an extended period. Remember that this is likely to be the part of your course where you have the greatest freedom to choose what you study. Even though you may not undertake the research, remember that you will need to spend a lot of time searching the literature and critiquing it, and drafting and redrafting a final form of words, so you need to be able to maintain your enthusiasm. At this point, you should also be clear about the aims and be able to justify why the topic is worth pursuing.

2. *What will fit your course requirements?* You need to familiarise yourself with the expectations of your institution about the format and scope of your research proposal. Do not underestimate the importance of this, since your overall aim is to complete your nursing degree and this will only happen if your research proposal meets the course requirements, however good it may be.

3. *What are you able to study?* There are several components to addressing what it is possible to study. First, what can you research ethically? You need to consider how your research might impact on your participants and other stakeholders, if you were actually to undertake it, even if you are only writing a proposal. This will need to be discussed in detail in the proposal, concentrating on ethical principles rather than simply saying 'ethical approval will be gained prior to commencing the research'. Second, what do you have the time and resources to study? An old adage for a research project is: 'Think about what you want to do. Halve it, then halve it again and you may still struggle to get it all done'. Although you must consider the logistics of the proposal, 'scientific' justifications for sample sizes and recruitment strategies will be more impressive than saying 'this is a small project so I can only interview four people'. Third, what can you get access to study? Many research projects will require you to gain access to participants and you need to consider how practical this is; this should be acknowledged in the proposal.

It is important that your research question is not so broad that it is unrealistic for you to be able to answer it, nor so narrow that it lacks sufficient substance. It is more common for students to have difficulties because their research questions are too broad, rather than too narrow. Students often write proposals with lots of aims and objectives, which in reality would be too complex to undertake. Discuss it fully with your supervisor but stick with one or two aims and two or three objectives at the most. A common pitfall that nursing students make is to state as an aim or objective that they want to change practice. This is laudable but unless the project is specifically designed to change practice, such as in an action research design, it is unlikely to change anything and the best you can hope for is to inform practice or make recommendations.

A traditional recommendation from research supervisors is to be wary of choosing research topics that have attracted recent media attention. The rationale for this is that you are likely to find a considerable amount of media coverage, but little research or academic writing. The danger is that the final dissertation or proposal will reproduce the generalisations and stereotyping presented in the media reports with little evidence from research studies or academic writing. However, some topics do have a reasonable academic literature.

Why formulate an overall research question?

A clear question forms your aims and objectives, drives your choice of methodology and methods, and if you were actually to undertake the research it would require you to write up how the question was answered in the discussion section.

So, it is important to formulate an overall research question because it will focus your choice of research design and your literature search. It is all too easy to find yourself going in several different directions during a literature search or to collect too much unfocused data and then become confused about what to include and what to leave out. A research question needs to be a full sentence, probably starting with the word 'What' and ending with a question mark.

You may find that you have more than one overall research question. Try to avoid that as it will be confusing; but if it is unavoidable, link them well to form an overall research project. If you find that you have two entirely separate research questions, you probably have two research projects and you need to decide which one you want to undertake.

Choosing your research approach and design: Quantitative and qualitative research

Once you have formulated an initial research topic, you need to consider which research approach and research methods to propose. As we discussed in Chapter 1, social research has traditionally been divided into quantitative and qualitative approaches. These approaches have different views about the nature of knowledge and different methods and priorities. Although this distinction is contested (Layder, 1993), it is commonly used and there is little evidence of it abating completely (Clark et al., 2021).

An example of a student project using a quantitative approach

Here is an example of a student research proposal using a quantitative approach.

Case study 3.1: Survey design using questionnaires

Varsha is a final-year student who is interested in her fellow students' experiences of their nursing education. She proposes to use questionnaires to study her fellow students' attitudes towards their professional training, particularly whether they feel it is preparing them for the realities of working as qualified nurses. She is interested in whether participants' responses differ according to year of study, age, gender and amount of pre-qualifying experience. For example, Varsha has a hypothesis that older students will report higher levels of confidence in their ability to practise and wants to test this out. See Chapter 6 on questionnaires for a full discussion of this example.

Some examples of student projects using qualitative approaches

Case study 3.2: Focus group

Christina is a child health nursing student on placement in a hospital ward. She is interested in interprofessional working when there are concerns about a child's welfare.

Christina decided that a focus group would be a good research method because it would enable her to hear a range of views and enable participants to interact with each other and challenge one another's views. Christina's focus is on participants' professional experience rather than their personal biographies and it would take much longer to conduct interviews that would produce a similar amount of data. The disadvantages of focus groups are that it can be difficult to arrange for a group of people to meet, and the possibility that some group members will not feel able to express their opinions.

Christina considered how to select her participants and how many focus groups to run. Eight staff members were interested in being involved and Christina contacted staff on a neighbouring ward and managed to recruit another eight staff members, which would enable her to run two focus groups.

Case study 3.3: Interviews

Victoria is a mental health student on placement in a voluntary sector mental health organisation. She is interested in how voluntary sector staff view work in partnership with statutory sector mental health organisations and would like to use qualitative interviews to explore this further.

Victoria must decide who to include in her sample. She considers that the most appropriate strategy would be purposive sampling, in which she selects participants who are most likely to yield useful information. This is often based upon factors such as the participant's knowledge, experience or role. She decides to interview two groups of voluntary sector staff, one working in her placement agency and another in a similar voluntary organisation in a neighbouring area. She will focus on staff members who are likely to experience partnership working as part of their everyday role.

Do I really have to discuss epistemology?

In the last two chapters we have discussed epistemology as the study of knowledge and what 'counts' as valid knowledge. We then discussed some of the main epistemological positions that have influenced quantitative and qualitative approaches. A common student question is whether it is necessary to talk about epistemology in your final dissertation or proposal. The extent to which you are expected to be explicit about your epistemological position depends upon whether you are completing an undergraduate or postgraduate degree and the requirements of your individual institution. Most postgraduate taught courses like Master's degrees require you to discuss in significant detail your epistemological position, while doctoral students would expect this to be a major element of their work. Undergraduate courses may not, but this varies between institutions. In undergraduate nursing programmes, it is likely that some discussion of the underlying philosophical issues surrounding a qualitative or quantitative approach will be an impressive feature of your work and is likely to score higher marks than if it is largely ignored.

Either way, the important point is to not be intimidated by the terminology, but to read around the different approaches and make sure the approach you choose is reasoned as it determines your data collection methods: the research question dictates the epistemological position, which indicates the methods of data collection and analysis, rather than the other way around. Students may think they want to 'do qualitative research because it's easier', but this may not be possible for some questions, like comparisons between treatments. If you are interested in whether one treatment works better than another you will need to measure something in order to show that, one way or another.

Imagine that your epistemological position, design, and research methods are like different items of clothing. For example, if you choose a qualitative approach with an interpretative epistemology then choose a highly structured questionnaire, this is similar to choosing clothes that clash with each other; they don't look right together. While each item may be acceptable individually, the combination does not work as they are incompatible, and would lead a tutor to suspect that you did not really understand what you were talking about. Making the different items match is an important part of making your proposal credible.

Moving from a research topic to a specific research question

For some research projects, the transition from having a research topic to formulating a specific research question is smooth and unproblematic. For others, it can take considerable time to narrow down the research topic and this is usually something that happens in parallel with developing the literature review. When you see how others have approached your research topic and the range of methodologies they have used, this is likely to focus your thinking.

Case study 3.4: Concept mapping

As Christina's interest is in safeguarding children, she wants to propose an investigation into how professionals work together when there are child welfare concerns. However, she is unclear how she is going to narrow this topic down to a research question.

Christina decides to use a concept map to identify the different angles from which she could approach this topic.

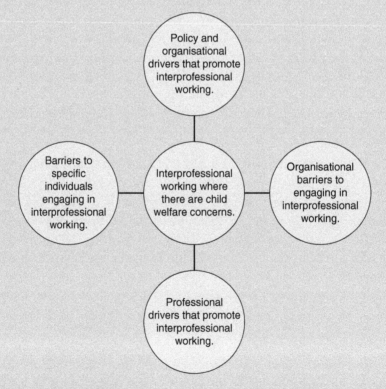

Figure 3.1   Initial concept map

Having completed her initial concept map (Figure 3.1), Christina decided that she was interested in identifying possible barriers to interprofessional working.

A useful tool or technique to aid this process is the concept map, which is a way of visually representing the different elements of your topic. Concept mapping allows you to think about your research topic because it helps you to break down your topic into its constituent parts and examine them in more depth.

Activity 3.1   Critical thinking

Write your research area at the centre of a piece of paper and map out the possible topics or angles from which you could approach it. Your aim is to move from a general topic area to a specific research question.

Comment

This can be useful to help you check your current understanding of your research topic. When you first do this, your concept map will represent your initial understanding of the topic. As you identify literature, you can update your concept map to create a visual representation of what material is available. You may find that there is a concentration of literature on particular topics, while other topics receive scant discussion. This will influence your choice and can be a useful subject for discussion in your literature review.

As this is your personal map, there is no outline answer at the end of the chapter.

Timetabling and resources

A coherent proposal gives a plan of what you intend to investigate and how you intend to go about it. It needs a timetable to show that you have considered all the steps necessary and allocated sufficient time to each. The key stages in a research proposal are as follows:

- ethics application and approval;
- literature review;
- recruitment;
- data collection;
- data analysis;
- writing up;
- dissemination.

Each of these needs to be allocated time. You may also want to include project meetings and time for writing your journal or reflective log. Proposals are generally planned with activities scheduled monthly rather than weekly. The time frame depends on your deadlines or coursework requirements; in reality this would depend on project funding, but for an undergraduate proposal this would not be a consideration. Designing a timetable can be done simply using a table in Microsoft Word (Figure 3.2): use the

Table function under the Insert tab, then shade the relevant months when the activities will be undertaken. This is a highly simplified example of how a proposal might be planned, and in reality, the stages would be more overlapping, with activities not necessarily carried out in such a delineated fashion. More complex and more interesting designs can be made using Gantt charts.

Activity	Sept	Oct	Nov	Dec	Jan	Feb	March	Apr	May
Ethics application and approval									
Literature review									
Recruitment									
Data collection									
Data analysis									
Writing up									
Dissemination									
Project meetings									
Reflective journalling									

Figure 3.2 Simple project planning using a Microsoft Word table

Resources

What will you need to help you to conduct the research? As a student writing a proposal, you are in the fortunate position of not having to think too much about the practicalities of this issue, but you may be asked to give an indication of the sorts of things you think you would need. In reality, the majority of research projects are entirely dependent on external funding from charities or government research organisations: they will not occur without it. Universities employ staff to conduct research as a result of getting external funding – they rarely fund studies from internal sources, and professors spend hours writing proposals and chasing funding bids. This is a highly competitive process, and careers are made as a result of obtaining large amounts of money. Nowadays, a system known as full economic costing (FEC) governs the estimates of sums of money included in bids that universities make. The University of Oxford site shows how they operationalise FEC (**https://researchsupport.admin.ox.ac.uk/costing-pricing**). Costing bids to external sources is a complex business and universities employ finance staff specifically for this purpose. Don't think about doing it yourself, as it's very difficult to get it right.

Activity 3.2   Critical thinking

In order to plan your resources, think through the sorts of things you think you would need for your project. Is this staff, computers, training, office space? Write down on a piece of paper what resources you will need.

There is a brief outline answer at the end of the chapter.

Dissemination

For a proposal you would not need to use any strategies for dissemination, but you might be asked to write about what you would do. There is an argument that conducting research purely for one's own purposes is unethical, and while undergraduate students are unlikely to have pressure put on them to publish their findings if they do undertake empirical research, postgraduate students will certainly be expected to do so. This is because findings contribute to a body of knowledge, even if it is a small contribution, and this body of knowledge may eventually become sufficient for changes in practice to be recommended. In general, dissemination would include publishing findings in journals. There is a distinction between good academic journals such as the *Journal of Advanced Nursing* and the *International Journal of Nursing Studies*, which have international reputations and readerships as publishers of research findings, and professional journals such as the *Nursing Times*, which aim to inform practice. It is quite hard to be published in academic journals, and you would need help from an experienced author to achieve this, but professional journals are usually slightly easier. As well as publishing in journals, you would need to write a project report. You could also present your findings at conferences. Although this may be scary at first, you get a great sense of achievement from it, and probably a couple of nights in a nice venue while you attend the conference.

Addressing ethical issues and research governance

All student research will need ethical approval from an appropriate ethics committee. Ethics committees are formal bodies that consider the ethical aspects of research studies and are constituted as part of the legal requirements of organisations, such as the NHS and universities. An important part of planning your research project is addressing ethical issues and following ethical governance processes. Each university has its own system of ethics committees and there are also similar processes within the NHS and other statutory agencies such as local authorities to protect patients, service users and staff from unethical research practices. As registrants, or potential registrants, with a professional body like the NMC, we also have a duty to abide by its code of conduct, and this overrides the fact that a student may be acting as a researcher: a nurse's first duty is to protect patients and clients at all times, and this should be acknowledged in proposals. If NMC registrants uncover issues of serious professional misconduct this must be passed on to the relevant authorities.

The NHS research ethics procedure is the most well known, and as a general rule any research proposal which intends to use NHS staff, patients/clients or facilities must consider submitting for ethical approval using the Integrated Research Application System (IRAS), although in many cases research simply accessing staff for their views about issues is unlikely to need NHS ethics approval. In March 2016, these processes came fully under the auspices of the Health Research Authority (HRA), whose remit, according to their website (**www.hra.nhs.uk**), is to protect and promote the interests of patients and the public in health and social care research, with a focus on making participants in health and social care research feel safe when they do so. There have been further revisions and simplifications to processes in 2018, when HRA Approval became HRA and Health and Care Research Wales (HCRW) Approval and now applies to all project-based research taking place in the NHS in England and Wales (other arrangements exist in Scotland and Northern Ireland); and in 2020 to align with the latest version of Governance Arrangements for Research Ethics Committees (GAfREC). Ethical approval and governance arrangements are dynamic processes and students must consult the relevant websites as things will change. Universities will have dedicated staff with remits to help and advise on ethical approvals via IRAS and these staff should be consulted at the earliest opportunity. From 2023, a pilot has been running to streamline research applications where NHS staff are participants.

There is a distinction to be drawn between ethical approval and governance approval. Broadly speaking, ethical approval means that a study raises sufficiently substantial ethical concerns about participants' autonomy, confidentiality, anonymity and personal safety that the proposal needs to be scrutinised and approved by a legal entity called a research ethics committee (REC). Governance approval means that the organisations in which the research is to take place give permission for it to go ahead because they are satisfied that the researchers have the capacity, capability and integrity to carry it out successfully (and without harm to participants). The HRA requires ethical approval for research involving any of the following:

- a clinical trial of an investigational medicinal product (CTIMP) (with the exception of phase 1 trials in healthy volunteers taking place outside the NHS);
- a clinical investigation or other study of a medical device;
- a combined trial of an investigational medicinal product and an investigational medical device;
- a clinical trial to study a novel intervention or randomised clinical trial to compare interventions in clinical practice;
- a basic science study involving procedures with human participants;
- a study administering questionnaires/interviews for quantitative analysis, or using mixed qualitative/quantitative methodology;
- a study involving qualitative methods only;
- a study limited to working with human tissue samples (or other human biological samples) and data (specific project only);
- a study limited to working with data (specific project only).

Research involving any of the following no longer requires NHS REC review:

- NHS staff recruited by virtue of their professional role;
- previously collected, non-identifiable tissue samples or information;
- acellular material, e.g. plasma or serum;

- healthcare market research;
- research involving premises and facilities (e.g. research undertaken by a university department on NHS premises, involving healthy volunteers not recruited as NHS patients and not subject to any legal requirements would not require review by an REC).

Applications for ethical approval in the NHS must go through its web-based IRAS, which is a unified system for applying for permission and approval for NHS research in the UK. In practice, IRAS has developed guidance for interpreting whether a study needs to come before its full ethics committee (REC) structure, and it draws a distinction between research, service evaluation and audit (NPSA, 2010). Its definition of research emphasises more experimental designs such as RCTs, which are evaluating new treatments or interventions with patients and clients, and there is also particular scrutiny of research where tissue samples are involved. As such, there is something of a dichotomy in this medical-model understanding of the term 'research', with its need to safeguard vulnerable patients and clients from the dangers of, for example, experimental medicines, compared to the understanding of research from a social science perspective, where 'research' means any type of inquiry where the intention is to study something by collecting data and creating new knowledge and/or understanding of that topic. This can work in the favour of nursing researchers because it can mean that their proposals may not actually need full REC approval through IRAS: projects evaluating the establishment of new services or roles within the NHS may be acceptable for academic awards and be considered 'research' in university departments but may be considered 'service evaluation' by IRAS. Students who are actually required to collect data should discuss this with their supervisors and use the HRA Decision Tool (see the useful websites section on pages 62–3). Some Master's students' proposals will not be eligible for ethical review in these processes. They recommend that Master's and PhD students complete their ethical review toolkit.

All proposals will require some work for them to be acceptable to any committee, and in your plan you need to allocate at least two or three months to get ethical approval based on submission deadlines, redoing and resubmitting the proposal before final approval. Two months is a bare minimum; three is more realistic. You cannot begin recruitment or data collection in any form until full ethical approval is obtained.

Permission to conduct a project

Regardless of whether your proposal would need to go to HRA ethical approval, you will need to obtain permission from each NHS site in which you plan to collect data, and this must be discussed in your proposal. Since March 2016, HRA has altered the processes required to gain what used to be called 'research governance approval' so that now, regardless of whether full REC approval is required, researchers apply for what is called permission to conduct a project, and this is also via the online IRAS. Before any data collection begins, students should contact the local research and development office in each NHS organisation where the research is planned and discuss with them exactly what is required and how they can help you with your application. In addition to this, researchers external to the NHS will need Honorary Contracts with the Trusts in which they plan to conduct research. This can take the form of a research passport, which covers all the human resource-type arrangements that a researcher would need to be accepted to work in the NHS.

University ethics approval

Universities have their own mechanisms for ethical approval, and students should check what these are and acknowledge them in their proposals. If your proposal would need to go for full REC approval via IRAS, when approved it may also need to go to your own university faculty ethics committee, at least so they know you have external approval via IRAS. Again, this will need to be factored into your timetable. If your proposal does not need full ethics committee approval, it will still need to be approved by your university who act as sponsor, and then submitted for permission via IRAS.

Non-NHS ethics approval

In 2005, the Government introduced the second edition of the Research Governance Framework (Department of Health, 2005) and this was updated in March 2023. It covers local authorities, and this has made a significant difference in research conducted in local authority areas, such as social work. Councils and local authorities have their own governance arrangements and committee structures, each of which differ slightly. Check out which procedures apply to you at the earliest stages of your research, as you need to consider and discuss them in your project proposal and allow sufficient time to address their requirements in your planning. The Social Care Institute for Excellence (SCIE) also has a research ethics committee, but this does not review student projects. In addition, remember that, increasingly, care is being provided in non-statutory settings, such as independent charities and third-sector organisations, which are not part of the NHS or local authorities. This is particularly the case in mental healthcare. Smaller organisations may not have ethics committees or formal governance arrangements but will need to have sight of, and give permission for, students' research to take place. They are likely to want to see ethical approval from a university committee before considering applications.

Activity 3.3   Evidence-based practice

List the ethical principles you think are important in research. Use your own language. Then, go to this British Medical Journal (BMJ) website on the Nuremberg Code (1947): **https://media.tghn.org/medialibrary/2011/04/BMJ_No_7070_Volume_313_The_**

Nuremberg_Code.pdf. Compare them with those established immediately after the Second World War. Next, go to the Declaration of Helsinki (World Medical Association, 2013) website at **www.wma.net/policies-post/wma-declaration-of-helsinki-ethical-principles-for-medical-research-involving-human-subjects** and do the same comparison.

Comment

The language is different, but the basic principles remain unchanged, if updated, between 1947 and 2013.

There is no outline answer at the end of the chapter.

Ethical principles

The formal consideration of ethical principles came after the Second World War when it came to light that Nazi medical staff had been torturing refugee camp inmates in the name of medical research. Following their convictions at the Nuremberg trials after the war, first the Nuremberg Code (1947) and then the declaration of Helsinki (last revised in 2013 – World Medical Association, 2013) enshrined ethical principles into medical research, and these have been adopted in all research fields.

Although different ethics committees have different practices and priorities, the core principles that ethics committees will be expecting you to address are as follows:

- Non-malevolence: have you taken all reasonable steps to protect your participants from foreseeable harm? For example, interviewing participants can be potentially upsetting and you need to think through how you can ensure they are supported. How will you ensure participants' confidentiality and anonymity?
- Informed consent: you will normally be required to provide written information to potential participants to enable them to make an informed choice. The NHS Health Research Authority provides examples of what information to provide **(www.hra-decisiontools.org.uk/consent/examples.html)**.
- Rights to refuse to participate or withdraw without prejudice: if participants do not want to be in the study or change their minds about allowing their data to be used after the event, what arrangements have you made to enable this? Is it clear that if potential participants refuse to take part, they will not be harmed in any way, including receiving less preferential treatment or care from service providers?
- Ethical data management: how will you anonymise your data and who will have access? How will you store the information that you gain? Have you taken reasonable steps to protect your participants from their data being lost? In some research studies you may be asked to provide a data management plan and consider the ethical governance of the data you collect. Your university will give you guidance on this if it is required.

Chapter summary

This chapter has looked at how you can plan the different stages of the research process. It began with some advice on how to choose your research area, narrow it down to a specific topic and then develop your research question. Techniques to help this process, such as using concept maps, were introduced.

The chapter then looked at how you can develop a plan for carrying out your research, including advice on drawing up a timetable. It looked at some of the resource issues that may arise and how you might anticipate them.

Finally, the chapter considered the ethics of research, and the issue of seeking ethical approval from your university or other body.

Activity: Brief outline answer

Activity 3.2   Critical thinking (page 54)

Exactly what you'll need depends on the study. In general, you could factor in:

- research assistant(s) – they will do all aspects of the study for you, from recruitment to data collection and analysis;
- computers – essential nowadays;
- office supplies – paper and other equipment;
- website – it is common for there to be a project website nowadays;
- travel expenses for you, your research assistant and participants;
- buy-out – do any of your participants need to be released from work to attend?
- professional or clinical services may be required if there are to be interventions – blood samples may need to be taken and analysed, or there may be more clinic visits;
- refreshments – cups of tea, biscuits and sandwiches may be offered as a thank you or because your interview sessions take place over mealtimes. Lunch for nurses and students is a reasonable 'perk' and an incentive to attend. Shopping vouchers may also work well.

Further reading

All the books listed below offer good coverage of project-planning issues.

Locke, LF, Spirduso, WW and Silverman, SJ (2014) *Proposals That Work: A Guide for Planning Dissertations and Grant Proposals* (6th edition). Thousand Oaks, CA: Sage.

Offredy, M and Vickers, P (2010) *Developing a Healthcare Research Proposal: An Interactive Student Guide.* Oxford: Wiley-Blackwell.

Punch, KF (2016) *Developing Effective Research Proposals* (3rd edition). London: Sage.

Robson, C (2007) *How To Do a Research Project: A Guide for Undergraduate Students.* Oxford: Blackwell Publishing.

Thomas, D and Hodges, ID (2010) *Designing and Planning Your Research Project.* London: Sage.

Walliman, NSR (2013) *Your Research Project: A Step-by-Step Guide for the First-Time Researcher* (2nd edition). London: Sage.

Useful websites

www.officetimeline.com/make-gantt-chart/excel

How to create a Gantt chart for a project plan using a Microsoft Excel spreadsheet.

www.crncc.nihr.ac.uk

Website of the National Institute for Health Research Clinical Research Network Coordinating Centre (NIHR CRN CC), which supports clinical research.

www.hra-decisiontools.org.uk/research

Health Research Authority Decision Tool. Guides you about whether your study requires submission to NRES or not.

https://encyclopedia.ushmm.org/content/en/article/the-nuremberg-trials

Website on the Nuremberg Trials.

www.hra.nhs.uk

Website of the Health Research Authority.

www.royaldevon.nhs.uk/about-us/research-and-development/

An example of the kinds of activities undertaken by a Foundation NHS Trust Research and Development Department. Contains a link to the Research Design Service (**www.rds-sw.nihr.ac.uk**), which can help with all aspects of project planning and funding applications. Many UK NHS Trusts have similar services, which may be accessed locally.

www.wma.net/policies-post/wma-declaration-of-helsinki-ethical-principles-for-medical-research-involving-human-subjects

World Medical Association website on the Declaration of Helsinki: Ethical Principles for Medical Research Involving Human Subjects.

Section 3

Using and critiquing research for your final-year project

Chapter 4

Using and critiquing qualitative research methods: interviews and focus groups

Chapter aims

After reading this chapter, you should be able to:

- understand how interviews and focus groups can be used as research methods;
- explain how to recruit and select participants for interviews and for focus groups;
- develop an interview schedule and understand the range of interview questions;
- be able to critique qualitative research using popular evaluation tools.

Introduction

This is the first of five chapters in this section that will introduce you to commonly used qualitative research methods and provide an overview of how interviews and focus groups can be understood and how that understanding can contribute to your final-year project or proposal. The emphasis in these chapters is in allowing you to choose the most effective method to use if writing a proposal, rather than in offering a guide of how to use the methods if you were actually undertaking projects for yourself. We will begin by talking about interviews, then move on to looking at focus groups. In the second part, we will discuss how to critique qualitative research methods using popular evaluation tools.

Interviews are one of the most popular qualitative research methods for nursing researchers and students and feel intuitively 'familiar' because of their use in everyday nursing practice. They are popular in the social sciences generally and are used in the majority of published qualitative research articles (Silverman, 2017). Many research studies use individual interviews to collect data, but focus groups are becoming increasingly popular, and rely on group dynamics to produce data on particular topic areas.

They are a form of interview, albeit one with a small group discussing ideas with a facilitator. Interviews and focus groups are examples of qualitative study designs. Broadly speaking, qualitative designs seek to understand and interpret the thoughts, feelings, behaviour, actions and cultures of individuals and groups. Their 'tools' are questioning, talking and analyses of texts, not numerical data (as would be present in a quantitative study design).

In this chapter, you will be asked to consider the advantages and disadvantages of these techniques and when it would be most appropriate to use them. Practical issues raised by their use will be emphasised through case studies and student-centred activities.

Interviews

The interest in interviews is not confined to nursing research. It can be argued that we live in an interview culture, in which we are constantly exposed to the idea that something valuable can be learnt by talking one to one with another person. Interviews are intuitively 'human', a face-to-face interaction that enables you to communicate with your participants in depth and offers the opportunity to follow up interesting responses. Interviews can enable people to tell their story and are particularly attractive when researchers want to explore people or communities that have traditionally been ignored, misrepresented or suppressed.

When should interviews be used?

Interviews are best used for research that focuses on the knowledge, values, beliefs and attitudes of participants. They are particularly good at helping participants to think through, consider and make explicit things that have previously been implicit. Robson (2016) argues that facts and behaviour are more easily obtained than beliefs and attitudes, though participants may experience memory lapses or bias so specific questions about things in the present or recent past are best. Questions about a participant's beliefs and attitudes are more complex because responses may be affected by the wording and sequence of questions, but the use of multiple questions and scales can help.

Interviews or questionnaires?

A common dilemma for students is deciding whether to use interviews or questionnaires. The advantages that interviews have over questionnaires is that interviews are good at examining complex issues and producing rich data and they enable participants to discuss sensitive issues in an open way without committing themselves in writing. The disadvantages are that interviews are more time-consuming to complete than questionnaires and it is more complex and time-consuming to analyse interview data.

Interviews or focus groups?

Another dilemma is whether to use interviews or focus groups. While focus groups are effective in accessing shared public knowledge, interviews are fruitful for more personal, biographical information. Interviews can be used in conjunction with focus groups where participants may disclose more sensitive information than they would in a group setting. See the section on focus groups in this chapter for a more detailed discussion.

Types of interview

Although there is a range of types of interview, the three main forms are structured, unstructured and semi-structured interviews.

Structured or standardised interviews

These are highly ordered and tightly designed interviews to collect data that can be quantified. You may have experienced a market research interview, in which multiple-choice questions with a fixed number of responses are used, but such interviews can also be used in the social sciences. Structured interviews have the strength that they are able to produce quantitative data in a clear, readily analysable form. However, they are less popular with students and nursing researchers because the closed nature of questioning does not give them sufficient scope to address more complex, rich, qualitative issues. Structured interviews are part of the quantitative survey research tradition and are similar to questionnaires, which will be discussed in Chapter 6. The remaining forms of interview are generally regarded as part of the qualitative research tradition and form the focus of this chapter.

Unstructured interviews

At the opposite end of the spectrum, unstructured interviews are very open and range from a single question to a list of topics. Sometimes students and nursing researchers consider unstructured interviews because they 'want the data to speak for itself'. Others consider it because they lack confidence in constructing a good *interview schedule* or are unsure about exactly what they want to focus on. The difficulty is that they then produce a number of interview transcripts that are very individual and often do not cover the same ground. This can be a strength for more experienced researchers who are confident in their abilities to analyse diverse and complex data but a real challenge to novice researchers. Consequently, unstructured interviews are best left to the more experienced researcher.

Semi-structured interviews

This is the classic structure for qualitative research in the social sciences and the most commonly used format in student research projects. In semi-structured interviews, the researcher develops a list of questions, known as an interview schedule.

However, there is some flexibility during the interview; for example, if a participant introduces a topic earlier than anticipated, the researcher can change the order of questions. The format is popular because it enables you to have sufficient structure to facilitate data analysis, while giving you sufficient flexibility to explore participants' responses in depth.

Recruiting and selecting participants

One of the most commonly asked questions is *how many people should I plan to interview?* There are usually methodological reasons, such as the achievement of data saturation, which will dictate sampling methods and hence recruitment in qualitative studies using interviews. These issues will need to be explained thoroughly in proposals and adhered to in any actual data collection. While it may also be true that logistical issues such as time constraints and course requirements will influence your recruitment, to list these will not impress supervisors or reviewers with your methodological knowledge and such explanations are best avoided. Consequently, discussing this with your supervisor or tutor is the best first step.

This chapter will focus on sampling strategies for using semi-structured or unstructured interviews within a qualitative approach, which is by far the most common approach used in student research projects. If you are planning to employ structured interviews using large sample sizes in a similar way to questionnaires, appropriate sampling strategies will be discussed in depth later.

In qualitative interviewing, the most common approach is non-probability sampling and the specific sampling strategies used are as follows.

Convenience sampling

Convenience sampling (sometimes known as *accidental sampling*) simply means selecting participants based upon the relative ease with which they can be contacted. When planning to use convenience sampling in qualitative research, researchers are not interested in how representative any participant is or whether the participant has particular knowledge or experience. Rather, they are looking for participants who are relatively easy to contact. While this is the least credible of sampling techniques, Clark et al. (2021) argue that this is far more prevalent than is often recognised in social science research and many quantitative studies and RCTs, in fact, use convenience sampling, despite the potential problems associated with it (Williamson, 2003).

Purposive sampling

Purposive sampling (otherwise known as judgemental sampling) is a procedure in which researchers choose participants who, in their judgement, are likely to yield useful information. This is often based upon factors such as the participant's knowledge, experience or role. Interviews are most successful when participants have significant experience in the research topic and are likely to want to discuss it. This is the most commonly used sampling method in student research projects and most writers on qualitative research based on interviews recommend it as the procedure of choice (Clark et al., 2021).

Theoretical sampling

Theoretical sampling is an approach, developed as part of grounded theory (Glaser and Strauss, 1967; Strauss and Corbin, 1998), which does not predetermine the number of participants that will be interviewed at the beginning of the study. Instead, researchers will carry on interviewing participants until 'saturation' has been achieved, where no significantly new data are being produced and the themes have been exhausted (Strauss and Corbin, 1998). It has been argued that purposive sampling and theoretical sampling are effectively synonymous (Lincoln and Guba, 1985; Brink, 2012).

Snowball sampling

Snowball sampling is a technique where the researcher selects a small number of participants and asks them to recommend other suitable people who may be willing to participate in the study. This is suitable when participants are difficult to identify and contact, such as sex workers or people who are homeless.

Quota sampling

Quota sampling is a procedure in which the researcher decides to research groups or quotas of people from specific subsections of the total population. Common categories are demographics such as age, gender and ethnicity, but could be related to the research topic. Quota sampling is rarely used in academic research, but it is used frequently in market research (Clark et al., 2021).

Case study 4.1: Qualitative interviews

Victoria is a nursing student on placement in a voluntary sector mental health organisation. She is interested in how voluntary sector staff view work in partnership with statutory sector mental health organisations and would like to use qualitative interviews to explore this further.

Activity 4.1   Critical thinking

Victoria must decide who to include in her sample. Now you have read through the previous sections, which approach do you think she would be most likely to choose?

There is a brief outline answer at the end of the chapter.

Ensuring that your data can be analysed

One of your main aims is to ensure that you show that you understand how to analyse data, and that the data will be readily analysable if you were to collect them. This cannot be overemphasised, because it is relatively easy to spend time and effort collecting significant amounts of interview data that you later discover are extremely difficult to analyse.

How easy it is to analyse your data depends mainly upon two factors. The first factor depends on how structured your interview will be, since the more structured the interview, the easier it will be to analyse the data you produce. However, a certain amount of flexibility may be appropriate for your research topic. The second factor is how diverse your participants are in terms of experience, role or other issues. One of the most common pitfalls is to choose a sample of participants with such a wide range of roles or backgrounds that the interview data are difficult to analyse. We will discuss qualitative data analysis in more detail in Chapter 5.

Developing an interview schedule

In your project proposal you may be asked to develop a schedule of questions, as this will show how you will go about collecting data which answer your research questions. Your interview schedule is a written plan of how you are going to structure the interview, including what questions you are going to ask and approximately in what order. In Chapter 3, we discussed how to develop research questions so it may be useful to revisit this. Remember that your study is seeking to answer a specific overall research question. When developing your interview schedule, your aim is to ensure that your overall research question is answered while promoting a natural flow of conversation that encourages your participants to talk in an open and relaxed way.

Do not be tempted to jot down a few vague ideas and hope that you can muddle through. Without a clear schedule of questions, it is likely that, if data were collected, the data would be muddled, take much longer to analyse, and not clearly answer the research questions you have decided upon.

During the initial stage of developing an interview schedule, it can be helpful to meet up with a few interested people to generate possible interview questions. Ideally, this would include at least one person who would fit the criteria for your sample because they may spot problems that others may miss. (This could be described as a 'pilot study'.) Likely people to invite could include your practice supervisor, placement colleagues and fellow students as well as any party interested in your specific research topic. You should also consider whether service users and carers could be useful in the design stages.

Once you have generated a range of possible questions in the group, take these away to work on them on your own. Review them and discard any that are clearly not relevant. Then divide them into two groups: 'need to know' and 'nice to know'. 'Need to know' questions are vital to answering your research question, while 'nice to know' questions are ones that you are simply curious about. Be honest and ruthless about this and you will probably be surprised by how many fall into the latter category, leaving you with a schedule of essential questions, which you have thought through and are confident about. It may be helpful to arrange another time to meet up with the group when you can test out the questions that you have selected and discuss the order in which they should be asked.

Activity 4.2   Decision making

Construct an interview schedule for Victoria (see the case study on page 69). First, construct a question, then think about five relevant questions, then identify which are essential and which are desirable.

There is a brief outline answer at the end of the chapter.

Using vignette questions

An interesting and useful form of questioning is the vignette, which is a simulation of real events depicting hypothetical situations. The most usual way of presenting information is through written material, but alternative formats, such as video material and cartoons, can be used. Vignettes present a scenario to participants, who are then asked about their attitudes, beliefs and responses. For example, in the case study Victoria could present a scenario in which there was a dilemma about inter-agency working. She could then ask participants how they would react in the scenario and explore the reasoning behind their choices.

The advantage that vignette questions have over more general questions is that they root the question in a specific situation. For example, if general questions are used to ask practitioners how they manage risk when accessing patients or clients, each may respond with broad comments that would be difficult to compare. If the same practitioners are presented with a specific scenario, they are all responding to the same information, so it would be easier to compare their responses. Vignette questions can be particularly effective when dealing with sensitive issues, since vignettes present a hypothetical scenario that can make it less confrontational than asking participants about their own experiences.

Vignettes can have more than one stage. For example, a scenario is presented, and participants are asked for their immediate responses. They are then presented with further information as the vignette develops and asked about their responses given the new information. This can be used to explore the effects of specific factors.

Advantages and disadvantages of interviews

Interviews have a number of advantages and disadvantages as a research method that you want to employ for your proposal. They may feel intuitively 'familiar' to you because you use them in your everyday nursing practice. You are more likely to have skills and experience of interviews than other research methods and are more likely to feel confident using them. Interviews enable you to access people's feelings and attitudes and allow you to probe for more detailed responses. Consequently, they provide richer and more in-depth data. They enable you to follow up interesting responses in ways that are not possible using other methods, such as questionnaires. If you are interested in participants' individual views and experiences, interviews are more likely to provide a setting that is conducive to openness than a focus group (unless the group is carefully constructed with friends or peers as participants) and will be useful as your proposal's method of data collection. Key disadvantages are the extent to which the researcher can 'lead' or bias responses, participants can be intimidated, responses can be misinterpreted, and participants may fail to turn up.

Recording the interview

By far the best practice is to record interviews, and this should be written into your proposal. Saying you'll use field notes that you write up after the interview will not give you the depth, immediacy or nuance that is required, and won't allow you to transcribe verbatim and quote participants. Recording interviews allows you to:

- give participants your full attention rather than dividing it between writing and listening;
- obtain a full record of the interview that you can make notes from and come back to.

Be aware though that your participant might be uncomfortable with recording or might be more wary of being open and honest.

The two options for recording your interviews are video or audio recording. Video recording captures non-verbal communication but is rarely used because it is so intrusive. Audio recording is generally regarded as good enough without being too disruptive. You can use either tape or digital audio recording.

Transcribing audio recording of interviews

Transcribing audio recordings of interviews is a time-consuming process. One hour of interview can take 2–6 hours to transcribe and the transcript can be 20–40 pages (Boyatzis, 1998). Although it may seem like just a boring administrative task, it is far more than that, and you need to acknowledge this in your proposal: analysis begins with basic listening to recordings to see patterns occurring. Transcribing provides a useful opportunity to continue this analysis before you begin the formal process of data analysis (see Chapter 5 for a detailed discussion of data analysis). However, this is an onerous task and students should consider software that automatically transcribes speech, which is available in Microsoft Word and Mac programs. Video-recording software such as Microsoft Teams and Zoom now have transcription software built in and these have become very accurate.

Researcher reflexivity

While quantitative research has traditionally used the concept of objectivity to seek to remove the researcher from the study through addressing issues of bias, qualitative research argues that this is neither possible nor necessarily desirable. In qualitative research, an alternative criterion for establishing trustworthiness is confirmability, which refers to the extent to which the data obtained from interviews are shaped by the participant rather than the personal interests, values, and biases of the interviewer (Lincoln and Guba, 1985). This requires you to be aware of what you bring to the task of interviewing your participants at multiple levels. At a practical level, this involves you being aware of how you may inadvertently shape the responses of your participants, e.g. by nodding enthusiastically when participants provide responses that you agree with and having neutral or negative body language when they make statements that you disagree with. At a deeper level, it is about your own reflexivity as a researcher, which is central to qualitative research.

The concept of reflexivity acknowledges that we bring our own thoughts, values and beliefs derived from our personal and professional background to our research. Viewed from a reflexive point of view, subjectivity is not a problem but an asset. For example, our experiences may sensitise us to aspects of a situation that others would overlook. But we need to be conscious of how our experiences may also mean that we are unaware of, or make assumptions about, other aspects of the situation. It is not possible for us to be free from assumptions, but reflexivity enables us to become aware of and explicit about these assumptions. To illustrate this, see the case study below.

Case study 4.2: Researcher reflexivity

Susan is a nursing student who is interested in undertaking qualitative interviews with nursing staff in an emergency department about managing patients who have injuries related to drinking alcohol. As she is developing the proposal, she has been keeping a reflexive journal.

(Continued)

(Continued)

In a journal entry, she reflected upon her own experiences and attitudes towards alcohol and how these may have influenced her approach. She reflected upon how her family tended to drink on family occasions and how she enjoyed this. She also reflected upon the attitude she had towards drinking in her peer group both as she grew up and in her current student group, where drinking was an essential part of her social life. She explored how this had shaped her attitudes towards alcohol, including her interest in the research topic itself.

She become worried that she was not 'objective' and thought that another student from a different background, e.g. someone who had grown up in a family where drinking alcohol was not acceptable, might approach the topic from a more objective perspective.

Activity 4.3   Critical thinking

Consider what we might learn about researcher reflexivity from the case history above. In particular:

1.   How might Susan's background influence how she approaches interviews with participants?
2.   To what extent do you think that the other student she envisaged would be more objective?

There is a brief outline answer at the end of the chapter.

Ethical data management

In 2018 the European Union implemented the General Data Protection Regulations (GDPR), and the UK passed a 2018 revised Data Protection Act (DPA) which supercedes the 1998 DPA. Broadly speaking, the GDPR tightens rules and regulations governing storage, sharing and usage of personal data by companies and organisations, sets higher penalties and establishes a more robust governance and reporting regime than previously. The GDPR applies across Europe and the UK DPA (2018) is an example of local implementation. Included in the UK Act is specific consideration of 'approved medical research', meaning studies have been approved by HRA and other bodies. The 2018 Act does not alter the requirements much compared with the 1998 version regarding research studies. Researchers handling personal information must comply with various principles and the Act gives participants rights over their personal information. Your proposal will need to address these issues and some suggestions concerning how this might be achieved are as follows.

You must comply with the Act in full or make the data completely anonymous so that the data now fall outside the Act's definition of personal data. This will be the case when it is impossible to identify the individuals from their data. This includes any other information held. An anonymous list with a separate key listing participants by a number or pseudonym will still not be completely anonymous under the terms of the Act, so you must anonymise data and not keep a record of who is who in the study. In this case, you can use the data without making arrangements to comply with the Data Protection Act because the data will no longer fall within the Act's definition of personal data.

You have a duty to ensure that participants' information is kept safe in a locked or otherwise secure location. Any papers must be kept in a locked filing cabinet and shredded when no longer required. Transcripts held as computer files should be password-protected so that the data are protected by a double layer of security: an initial password verification when logging in and a password for each individual folder or file. You can also encrypt data: this is even more secure. When deleting electronic data, it is not enough simply to press delete and empty the recycle bin as this only removes the file name; the data will still be accessible to a knowledgeable third party. Instead, data must be destroyed securely or 'shredded'. Software for password protecting and encrypting data is already loaded in Windows PCs and Apple Macs. For shredding folders and files, you will need to download tools for this depending on your software and you should consult the relevant support websites for this.

Focus groups

This section introduces you to another commonly used research method that may inform your proposals: focus groups. Although group interviews have a long history in market research and were used to evaluate propaganda during the Second World War, it is only relatively recently that focus groups have become more popular as a research method in the social sciences. This can be contrasted with anthropological techniques, which have been around for over 100 years.

Focus groups are versatile and have been used for a wide range of topics. For example, focus groups have been used to research student nurses' experiences of collaborative learning in practice placements (Williamson et al., 2020), the understanding of elder abuse in residential settings (Myhre et al., 2020), understanding and young people's experiences of gangs in London (Whittaker et al., 2020).

Defining focus groups

A focus group is a group of individuals selected to provide their opinions on a defined subject, facilitated by a moderator who aims to create an open and relaxed environment and promote interaction between participants. Rather than an interview with a number of participants giving their views, focus groups enable discussion between participants. Such discussions can enable participants to explore and challenge each other's views and can result in people clarifying and changing their views, and this interaction could be an important factor in deciding to choose them for your proposal.

Combining focus groups with other research methods

Focus groups are often used on their own, but can be combined with other research methods, such as surveys or interviews. You may want to use focus groups before a survey to provide an overview and test the range of opinions, which will be used in questionnaire construction.

Interviews can be used in conjunction with focus groups where participants may disclose more sensitive information than they would in a group setting. Whereas focus groups are effective in accessing shared public knowledge, interviews are fruitful for more personal, biographical information. For research topics that require both forms of knowledge, combining both methods can be productive.

Research summary: Combining focus groups and interviews

Michell (1999) conducted a longitudinal study of teenage lifestyles that followed a cohort of 11- and 12-year-olds over time. She sought to understand how changing peer group structures influenced health behaviours. She used a combination of focus groups and interviews to examine teenage relationships, particularly the 'pecking order' in peer relationships.

Michell found that there were three identifiable groups: 'top' or popular girls, 'middle' girls and marginalised or 'bottom' girls. One of the most interesting insights was the difference between the data revealed in the focus groups compared to the interviews. For 'top' and 'middle' girls, there was little difference between what they said in the focus groups and what they said in the interviews. For marginalised or 'bottom' girls, the picture was quite different. While 'top' and 'middle' girls acknowledged their own status in the focus groups, 'bottom' girls did not and were often quieter and sometimes silent. 'Bottom' girls only acknowledged their status in individual interviews and discussed their difficulties in school and often at home.

This difference was only noted in 'low status' girls. By contrast, Michell found that 'low status' boys responded in focus groups and interviews in similar ways. She described them as *either silent or at best monosyllabic in both settings or were silly and disruptive, relating wildly implausible anecdotes about violence and drug use, etc.* (Michell, 1999, page 46).

This interesting study provides a useful insight into the limitations of focus groups for topics that require subjects to discuss both public, shared knowledge and personal, biographical information. Combining both methods enabled the researcher to access both forms of knowledge successfully.

Advantages and disadvantages of focus groups

Focus groups enable you to gain a range of opinions about a topic in a fairly easy and reliable way. They can produce significant amounts of data focused on a specific topic and are less time-consuming than interviews. They provide an opportunity for participants to express a range of opinions and challenge and interact with one another in an open environment. Participants can explore and develop their opinions through interactions with others and provide insights into complex behaviours. They are often seen as more democratic in that there may be six or eight participants but only one researcher, who is therefore 'outnumbered', and the power differential between researcher and participants is less than in a one-to-one setting. Finally, they are more accessible than other research methods for people with literacy difficulties or for people who do not have English as a first language.

Arranging times and venues for a group of people to meet can be complex and demanding, however, and requires you to engage in considerable negotiation and coordination. Some group members may feel unable to voice their opinions because they feel less confident or less powerful or feel their opinions may be unacceptable to other group members. Recruiting group members from similar backgrounds and a skilled moderator can significantly reduce these risks. The nature of the group context may mean participants do not discuss personal experiences and histories in as much depth or detail as individual interviews. Recording and transcribing can be time-consuming and complex; for example, identifying the contribution of different participants from an audio tape when they have similar voices. Finally, focus groups offer less control over the discussion than an interview.

When not to use focus groups

There are a number of circumstances when focus groups are best avoided, and you need to think these through carefully before proposing them in your project. First, when boundary issues may become too complex; for example, participants have complex relationships with each other that involve potential role conflicts. Second, when you are seeking to learn about the individual history and biography of participants. Third, when you are seeking to make statistical generalisations about a wider population. Fourth, where it would be extremely difficult to bring participants together at a certain time and venue. Finally, if you are relatively new to research, avoid using focus groups to discuss issues that are likely to be very distressing to participants. Focus groups have been successfully used for sensitive topics, but require considerable experience and skills in moderation, although don't let this put you off planning them in your work.

Selection and recruitment issues

There is considerable debate about the 'ideal' size for a focus group. Although groups of 8–12 are thought desirable for market research purposes, social research usually uses smaller group sizes, often 6–8 participants (Krueger and Casey, 2015). It can also depend upon how aware the participants are of the topic – larger groups are necessary when participants have low levels of awareness, whereas smaller groups enable highly aware participants to discuss the topic in detail. Drop out (usually 10–20 per cent) occurs and must be planned for.

When deciding how many focus groups to plan, the general consensus for large-scale projects is that it is best to plan three or four focus groups with any one type of participant, that is, three different groups of nurses (Krueger and Casey, 2015).

Student research proposals often plan one or two focus groups. Different university supervisors or tutors will have different opinions on this, but one to three groups usually provide sufficient useful and stimulating data to analyse.

'Naturally occurring' and 'stranger' groups

There are two types of focus group: a 'naturally occurring' group and a 'stranger' group. The naturally occurring group comprises participants who know each other in another role, such as a work team or support group. The stranger or assembled group comprises people who do not know each other but have a similar background or similar experiences. Neither is regarded as being 'better' than the other and your choice depends upon your research proposal.

A potential issue when using naturally occurring groups is the possibility of 'groupthink', although this can occur in any group. This is the tendency for dissenters in groups to suppress their opinions and for the group to reach a consensus quickly without critically considering the alternatives to avoid conflict (Janis, 1982). This can be challenged and explored by a sensitive moderator and can lead to rich and interesting data.

If your research focuses on the 'taken for granted' assumptions underlying a topic, a stranger group may have the advantage that participants are likely to spend more time explaining their reasoning. Stranger groups are popular in market research for this reason, whereas naturally occurring groups are more common in student research.

Recruiting and selecting participants

You need to outline your recruitment strategy in your proposal. Participants for a natural group can be recruited in a number of ways. One of the easiest ways is to use existing networks; for example, designing a poster or e-mail to be distributed, or being invited to meetings to explain your research. Asking a key figure to distribute information can be effective, provided participants do not feel under pressure to participate. Some research projects offer incentives, such as gift tokens, but providing refreshments and food can be equally successful.

In your plan, you should aim to minimise recruitment bias rather than achieve generalisability. Recruitment bias occurs when groups do not reflect the diversity of potential participants. For example, planning a focus group evaluating a service by approaching the manager for details of potential participants is likely to generate a list of service users who feel positively about the service. It is difficult to eliminate this entirely; for example, a poster invitation will still attract people who normally get involved in such activities. Any method has strengths and weaknesses, and these must be acknowledged in proposals. If you are seeking to be able to generalise statistical findings to a much wider population, a quantitative approach such as surveys with a larger sample size using the relevant statistical tests is necessary.

Homogeneous or heterogeneous group?

Although there is debate whether focus groups should be homogeneous (similar) or heterogeneous (dissimilar), most researchers prefer a homogeneous group who share a background or experiences that are the focus of the discussion. Having a homogeneous group is advantageous because it can help to ensure that participants feel able to speak freely and lead to data that are more straightforward to analyse (Krueger and Casey, 2015). Heterogeneous groups are particularly problematic where there are power differentials between participants because apparent consensus may not reflect the real views of all members (Krueger and Casey, 2015).

If participants are selected to be placed in groups of similar people, known as 'segmenting', the most common categories in large-scale research projects are gender, race, age and social class. For nursing students, the categories are more likely to be related to role or grades within particular roles – for example, service users or patients, critical care nurses, Band 5 and 6 nurses, healthcare assistants and assistant practitioners and so on – though the previously mentioned factors should also be considered where relevant.

Case study 4.3: Planning a focus group

Stephen is on placement in a large, acute-sector NHS hospital Trust. He is interested in nurses' views on improving patient care in a surgical ward.

Stephen decided that a focus group would be a good research method because it would enable him to hear a range of views and for participants to interact with each other and challenge each other's views. His focus was on participants' professional experience rather than their personal biographies and it would take much longer to conduct interviews that would produce a similar amount of data. The disadvantages are that it can be difficult to arrange for a group of people to meet, the risk of 'groupthink' and the possibility that some group members do not feel able to express their opinions.

Stephen considered how to select his participants and how many focus groups to run. There are 50 full- and part-time nurses in the team, a senior matron and her three deputy managers. Sixteen staff members were interested in being involved and Stephen decided against involving the manager and deputies because the power differential might make it difficult for participants to speak openly. He decided to run two focus groups, with qualified nurses in one group and unqualified ones in the other, to gain perspectives from the different staff groups and to prevent the unqualified staff from feeling inhibited by their 'seniors'.

Discussion guides

A discussion guide is a list of topics or questions that you produce for yourself as the moderator to guide the conversation in a focus group. It is likely that you'll need to include this in your proposal. Assuming a two-hour focus group, it is realistic to ask 8–12 questions, depending upon the type of question (Krueger and Casey, 2015). The group nature of the discussions means that fewer questions are asked than in individual interviews.

A discussion guide should have a clear structure and will include a range of different types of question:

1. Introduction: summarises the research topic briefly, confidentiality, recording and ground rules. For example:

    o   only one person speaking at a time;
    o   no side conversations among neighbours;
    o   everyone participating, with no one dominating;
    o   keep it as brief as possible.

2. Warm-up questions: these aim to help participants feel comfortable with speaking in the group and are usually short, factual questions that every participant responds to. Ensuring that everyone makes an initial statement can also reduce the risk of groupthink.

3. Introductory questions: these introduce the topic and provide a context, encouraging participants to think about the key topics.

4. Key questions: these are the principal questions that directly address your research question. Up to half of the questions will be in this category.

5. Closing questions: these enable the moderator to check their understanding of what has been said, to enable participants to provide a summary view and to provide an opportunity for any issues not discussed to be addressed. Krueger and Casey (2015) identify three questions in this category:

    o   The 'all-things-considered' question: used to clarify the final position of participants on the topics discussed and their relative importance (e.g. 'all things considered, what is the most important issue we have discussed here today?'). This is particularly important if participants have changed their views and if they have discussed relatively minor issues more frequently than more important issues.
    o   The summary question: the moderator attempts to summarise the discussion and asks whether it is a fair synopsis.
    o   The final question: having summarised the discussion, the moderator asks whether anything has been overlooked or whether participants want to add anything that they haven't previously said. Ask this with ten minutes left rather than at the very end, when participants may want to finish on time.

The analogy of a funnel is often used to describe the process of each focus group, starting with a less structured general discussion leading to a more structured discussion of specific topics. This allows the first part of the group to concentrate on participants' own perspectives on the topic and the second part to focus on the interviewer's specific interests in the topic.

Organising pilot focus groups is more difficult than pilot interviews, but you can get feedback that can significantly improve a discussion guide. The two best stages to involve other people are the initial stage of generating possible questions and the final stage of developing your discussion guide.

Case study 4.4: Developing a discussion guide

Stephen developed his discussion guide by involving his practice supervisor and a staff member from another team to generate some ideas for questions. Using a flipchart and pen, they spent 30 minutes generating as many questions as possible. He took these questions away and redrafted them, ensuring they were in the right sequence. He took them back to his practice supervisor and colleagues and they provided useful feedback.

It is unlikely that you'll need to say much about the role of the group moderator in a proposal, but the moderator's function is:

* to create an open and relaxed environment and promote interaction between participants;
* to promote the involvement of all participants without allowing particular individuals to dominate.

Having a colleague or fellow student who can assist you is essential, and this should be acknowledged in your proposal resources. As well as helping you to welcome participants and other practical support, they can take field notes, as it is virtually impossible to moderate well and take notes simultaneously. A debriefing session will help to clarify your ideas after the group ends.

It is unlikely that you'll need to say much about managing the group in a proposal, but key points are:

* a focus group is not a therapy or support group;
* its purpose is to gather data for your research project;
* try not to let groups become side-tracked with issues that are important to them but are not relevant to the research.

Case study 4.5: Stephen's focus group

It is the day of Stephen's first focus group, and one person is off ill, and another can't get away from the unit. This still leaves six people and Stephen has decided to go ahead. A colleague has agreed to act as assistant moderator, taking notes.

The group starts well, with participants writing down and then discussing their first impressions of the issues. When Stephen asks them about improving patient care, one participant states the whole team is already overworked, particularly as there is an unfilled vacancy. There is general unrest in the group and one participant starts whispering to another. The conversation turns to feeling overworked and undervalued in the service.

Activity 4.4   Reflection

If you were Stephen, how would you respond to this situation in your role as moderator?

There is a brief outline answer at the end of the chapter.

Recording and transcribing

Video recording would be ideal from a data-gathering perspective but is likely to be too intrusive for participants and the equipment is unlikely to be available. Audio recording is the most common compromise, enabling a recording to be kept while not being too intrusive.

There are a range of choices when writing up recordings, depending upon the rigour of your analysis and the time you have available:

- A full transcript: a verbatim transcript is produced and used alongside notes taken during the focus group and afterwards. For some forms of analysis, such as conversational analysis, transcripts should include every aspect of the conversation, including pauses and all verbal communication.
- Tape-based analysis and shortened transcript: a transcript is produced, but it covers the points made rather than being a verbatim account.
- Note-based analysis: this relies mainly on notes, a debriefing session and summary comments made at the end of the focus group. The session is taped but the tape is used to verify specific quotes.
- Memory-based analysis: notes can be consulted but most of the write-up is based upon recall.

Best practice is to fully transcribe the tape recordings and you should propose this in your plan. However, it may be acceptable to propose a lesser arrangement if focus groups are planned as a preliminary or exploratory measure for other research methods, such as surveys.

Critiquing qualitative research studies

In the preceding sections we have outlined key concepts in relation to using the main qualitative research methods, namely focus groups and individual interviews. In this section, we will discuss how to critique qualitative research methods using a range of popular evaluative tools. Critiquing, or critical appraisal, of qualitative research studies is about more than reading them and summarising them in any assignment; it is about deconstructing them and showing that you understand them and whether they have been conducted well or badly. Anyone can reproduce chunks of text from a study to another, but the point is to show that you have gone deeper than that. There are many tools that help you to read papers and make sense of them. A relatively easy tool comes from CASP available here: **https://casp-uk.net/casp-tools-checklists**. There are relevant ones for qualitative research, RCTs, case-control studies, cohort studies and systematic reviews, amongst others. The way to use them is to read the paper through once, then read it again with the CASP tool in front of you and make notes as you go.

In this chapter we have discussed qualitative research and so we will use the qualitative CASP checklist. There are ten questions, and you can answer Yes, No or Can't Tell, to the question. Each question has some hints about what is relevant.

It maybe that, when reading the paper with the checklist, most of the questions can be answered Yes. That is fine. In critical appraisal you are not necessarily looking for faults, although you may find some. You can still critically appraise an excellent paper by saying why it is so good and making reference to supporting research methods' literature to do so. However, when you find yourself answering No or Can't Tell, this is your 'ammunition' in the sense that the checklist is pointing you towards where you need to elaborate and expand on the areas listed.

For example, on the qualitative CASP checklist, question 6 is:

> Has the relationship between researcher and participants been adequately considered?

We have already discussed what is meant by reflexivity in this chapter. It is important and that is what this question is asking you to focus on. Why is it so important? It is about the researchers acknowledging their positions in relation to the research. What are the implications if it is not discussed? We cannot be sure that the researchers have been totally clear about how their views might have clouded their interpretations; they may have introduced bias and so the findings must be interpreted with caution. Consider the following CASP checklist hints:

- If the researcher critically examined their own role, potential bias and influence during (a) formulation of the research questions and (b) data collection, including sample recruitment and choice of location.
- How the researcher responded to events during the study and whether they considered the implications of any changes in the research design.

So, the hints are asking you to focus on just those features of reflexivity that we have identified as important. This construction of an argument about a paper based on critical appraisal will take time, wide reading and demonstrating an understanding of key research terminology. It is a bit like learning a new language. Stick at it and it will be rewarding. You can repeat the process for each of the ten CASP questions. Take notes, look up terminology and piece together your arguments.

Chapter summary

This chapter has introduced you to the key features of interviews as a research method and has provided some pointers about how to critically appraise papers that use these qualitative methods by using the CASP tool. You have considered when it would be most appropriate to use interviews compared to alternative approaches, such as questionnaires and focus group analysis. After studying the different types of interview, you examined some of the key issues around recruiting and selecting participants and applied this to a student case study.

This chapter has also looked at how to develop an interview schedule and understand the range of interview questions that are available to you. You reviewed the functions of different types of questions, paying particular attention to questions to avoid. A learning point from this chapter has been the importance of preparation, as careful thought at the early stages can save valuable time in the later stages.

Despite the challenges involved, interviewing is a popular and rewarding research method. It enables you to gain rich and complex data about people's knowledge, experiences, views, and attitudes. You have seen in this chapter that careful preparation can avoid the common pitfalls and help you to produce a research project that is well designed, interesting, and useful.

Focus groups are an increasingly popular research method that has been used to study a wide range of issues. They can be used as a stand-alone method or combined with other research methods, such as interviews or surveys.

Focus groups have a range of advantages and disadvantages. They enable you to gain a range of opinions in a fairly easy and reliable way and can produce significant amounts of data focused on a specific topic. They are less time-consuming than interviews and are more accessible than other research methods for people with literacy difficulties, people whose first language is not English and for traditionally marginalised groups. However, they can be difficult to arrange and recording and transcribing can be complex and time-consuming.

Focus groups can be either naturally occurring groups or stranger groups. Each has its strengths and weaknesses, and neither is inherently better. Focus groups in social research tend to be smaller than in market research, often involving six to eight participants. While large-scale studies involve three or more focus groups per category of participant to exhaust a topic, student research commonly involves one or two groups.

Different methods of recording focus groups were examined.

Activities: Brief outline answers

Activity 4.1   Critical thinking (page 70)

Victoria does not need to use convenience or snowball sampling because she has a number of potential participants who she can contact relatively easily. Since she is not using grounded theory to analyse her data, theoretical sampling is not necessary and quota sampling is rarely used in academic research, except in grounded theory. The most appropriate sampling strategy would be purposive sampling, in which she selects participants who are most likely to yield useful information. This is often based upon factors such as the participant's knowledge, experience or role. She decided to interview two groups of voluntary sector staff, one working in her placement agency and another in a similar voluntary organisation in a neighbouring area. She will focus on staff members who are likely to experience partnership working as part of their everyday role.

Activity 4.2   Decision making (page 71)

1.   Construct a research question for Victoria: 'How do voluntary sector mental health staff view partnership working with statutory organisations?'

2.   Think of five questions which she might ask workers that would support that research question by allowing participants to talk about the issue and give her relevant data. Examples might include the following:

     o   Tell me a bit about your relationship with staff in the statutory sector?

     o   Tell me a bit about your relationship with organisations in the statutory sector?

     o   What are the good things about working with the statutory sector?

     o   What are the bad things about working with the statutory sector?

     o   How could you and your organisation improve your working relationships with the statutory sector?

3.   The first four questions are essential and the last desirable, as the research question is about how voluntary sector mental health staff view partnership working with statutory organisations rather than changing that relationship.

Activity 4.3   Critical thinking (page 74)

1.   When Susan interviews participants, she may find that she inadvertently agrees slightly too enthusiastically when participants take an 'alcohol isn't that bad, we all do it' attitude, while being silent or appearing disapproving when participants criticise patients for drinking any alcohol at all.

2.   From the perspective of reflexivity in qualitative research, neither student would be 'objective'. Each would simply bring different experiences, values and beliefs to the research topic. Rather than seeking to attain perfect 'objectivity', the aim of reflexivity is for researchers both to be aware of what they bring and to be open and explicit about this in the research process.

Activity 4.4   Reflection (page 82)

The risk is that the discussion is likely to get side-tracked into a general discussion about staff shortages and the additional work pressures this causes. While this is important to the team, it is not productive for the research question.

If participants become side-tracked with an issue that they feel is important for them, but which is tangential to your topic, you need to bring them back to the research questions. It is important to do this sensitively, so participants do not feel censured. For example, you could say, 'That's an important topic, but I would like to hear more about …'. If participants continue, it is important to persist; for example, saying 'Perhaps we can come back to that later, but X made an interesting point and I would like to hear more about …'.

When groups get side-tracked by other issues, one thing to consider is whether the question is quite difficult or challenging for participants and they are avoiding responding to it. If the group continues to get side-tracked, it can be helpful to ask directly whether the question is difficult to respond to. Expressing this openly enables participants either to address the question directly or to explore the reasons why it might be a difficult topic to talk about. Either way, it will produce useful data that are relevant to the research question.

Further reading

On interviews

Kvale, S and Brinkmann, S (2014) *InterViews: Learning the Craft of Qualitative Research Interviewing* (3rd edition). London: Sage.

The third edition of a classic text on interviews, which places interviewing firmly within the qualitative tradition. Chapter 7 provides a practical overview of the interview process, while the early chapters address key theoretical issues.

Mason, J (2017) *Qualitative Researching* (3rd edition). London: Sage.

A solid and well-written textbook that combines practical considerations with detailed consideration of theoretical and methodological issues. Chapter 4 on qualitative interviewing is particularly clear and helpful.

On focus groups

Krueger, RA and Casey, MA (2015) *Focus Groups: A Practical Guide for Applied Research* (5th edition). Thousand Oaks, CA: Sage.

An excellent introductory text giving sound, practical advice.

Sim, J (1998) Collecting and analysing qualitative data: issues raised by the focus group. *Journal of Advanced Nursing*, 28 (2): 345–352.

A helpful article about data analysis issues for focus groups.

Useful websites

https://gdpr.eu/what-is-gdpr/

Information website about the GDPR.

www.gov.uk/data-protection

UK government website on the Data Protection Act (2018).

Chapter 5 Analysing qualitative data

Chapter aims

After reading this chapter, you should be able to:

- understand the concept of thematic analysis of qualitative data;
- use thematic analysis to inform strategies for planning a proposal;
- be aware of the particular issues that apply to data gathered from focus group discussions;
- use your understanding of data analysis to critique qualitative research findings.

Introduction

In this chapter, we look at approaches to data analysis, examining the analysis of data from interviews and focus groups. We will start from the perspective of choosing potential strategies when planning a proposal and will refer to aspects that are important when critiquing research findings.

Data analysis is the process that researchers use to make sense of the information collected and in searching for what lies below the surface content in order to grasp how to understand the often complex story that their data tell. Qualitative data analysis can be likened to skills that we use every day in our nursing practice: when we meet a new patient or client, we seek to understand that person's unique situation. When we have met a number of them in similar situations, we start to see patterns in what they tell us. We try to identify similarities and differences and start to see links and relationships between the different aspects of their experiences. This helps us to build up our understanding of those experiences that can be helpful for new service users that we meet.

Qualitative data analysis also involves new skills and techniques, which can seem daunting and confusing at first: it is not helpful to see it as a highly technical, almost mystical process, but neither is it true that findings will be obvious in the mass of data collected. Developing themes and writing these in a coherent manner which addresses the aims and objectives of a study is in itself a skill, which can be developed and is best understood in the context of existing methods which give an element of structure and robustness to the analysis.

Analysing qualitative data

The term 'data analysis' may provoke images of number crunching and statistical tests. However, in qualitative research, the data being analysed are words. These are the words of participants during interviews and focus groups. It is possible to analyse visual material or observational data, but these are specialised areas not covered in this book. In qualitative research, data analysis is the fascinating process of making sense of what people have said, identifying patterns and understanding meanings. Miles and Huberman (1994) capture the inherently interesting nature of this process:

> *Qualitative data are sexy. They are a source of well-grounded, rich descriptions and explanations of processes in identifiable local contexts. With qualitative data one can preserve chronological flow, see precisely which events led to which consequences, and derive fruitful explanations.*

(Miles and Huberman, 1994, page 1)

While you have to be consistent and systematic in how you interpret your data, the complexity of how to interpret meaning means that rigid rules for data analysis are rarely possible or indeed helpful. Qualitative data analysis is a contested area, with no universally agreed rules and many different interpretations in a variety of authoritative textbooks. There are, however, broad guidelines and applying them requires researchers to exercise judgement and make explicit decisions. This section will concentrate upon data collected from interviews and focus groups.

Alternative approaches to analysing qualitative data

There is a wide range of approaches to analysing qualitative data to choose from, coming from different research traditions. It is important to choose an approach to data analysis that is compatible with your research question and overall research approach. Some methods of data analysis require you to adopt a specific research approach, such as grounded theory and interpretative phenomenological analysis (IPA), while others are compatible with a wide range of research approaches, such as thematic analysis. In this chapter, grounded theory and thematic analysis will be discussed as two of the most common approaches. Grounded theory will be briefly outlined but the primary focus will be on thematic analysis as a sound and robust approach for new researchers.

Grounded theory

Grounded theory was developed in the late 1960s as qualitative data analysis was becoming more widely accepted (Glaser and Strauss, 1967). It was developed as a systematic way of analysing data that sought to address concerns at that time that qualitative research did not meet the standards of validity and reliability expected in quantitative research. Grounded theory is an approach to research that emphasises the importance of generating new concepts and theoretical frameworks from data. The name 'grounded theory' captures its aim of seeking to generate theory that is grounded in the careful analysis of data, rather than the testing of existing theory. There are different schools within grounded theory, starting with Glaser and Strauss (1967) developing different versions of grounded theory after their original publication, and no single version predominates.

Grounded theory is not just a method for analysing data but a whole approach to research. Key concepts in grounded theory are constant comparison, theoretical sampling and theoretical saturation. Data collection and analysis happen alongside one another and data are analysed as they are collected in a continuous process of constant comparison. Theoretical sampling is an approach in which sampling evolves as the research develops rather than being predetermined. For example, early data collection and analysis in an observational study about dignity on hospital wards may suggest that 'privacy' is an important category so the researcher can seek opportunities to observe settings where patient privacy is central. Early sampling is usually directed towards having a wide variety of data, which is progressively narrowed as the analysis develops. This continues until new data do not provide any new insights, the point known as theoretical saturation.

Grounded theory has been subjected to a number of criticisms. The claims by grounded theory that it generates theory have been disputed. It is argued that, in many instances, what is generated are findings that are specific to particular localised settings rather than formal theory, though they may have wider applicability. Grounded theory discourages researchers from conducting extensive literature reviews before starting data collection because this can lead to findings that are grounded more in the existing literature rather than the data. However, the ability of researchers to suspend their existing knowledge until the later stages of analysis has been questioned more recently and it is now generally accepted that theory-free observation is unrealistic (Clark et al., 2021).

Understanding thematic analysis

Thematic analysis is a very common model for analysing qualitative data (Clark et al., 2021). We will introduce you to this clear and systematic way of analysing your data based upon a model of thematic analysis developed by Braun and Clarke (2006, 2013).

Thematic analysis has been defined as *a method for identifying, analysing and reporting patterns (themes) within data* (Braun and Clarke, 2006, page 79). It is a foundational method that offers core skills that are useful for other forms of qualitative analysis. Thematic analysis is a flexible approach that is compatible with different epistemological approaches. We have previously discussed the distinction between positivist/realist and interpretivist/social constructionist approaches (see Chapter 1) and thematic analysis can be used with both approaches.

The process of thematic analysis

Braun and Clarke (2006, 2013) outline a six-stage model for the process of analysing data. Before we look at this in detail, it is important to define some key terms. *Data set* refers to the total data collected that will be used in the analysis. *Data item* refers to a particular interview or focus group, while *data extract* refers to a passage that has been taken from a data item such as a quote from an interview. Research reports should contain some information about the processes used to analyse data and the information below will help you to understand what they should have done and therefore identify any potential critique of their methods.

Phase 1: Becoming familiar with the data

Data analysis should begin with the immersion of the researchers in the data by reading through all the transcripts at least once, which will enable them to become sensitised to the material and develop an awareness of the whole data set. Where one researcher has collected and transcribed the data him/herself, he/she will already have a good level of prior knowledge of the key issues in the data set but seeing it written down can enable the person to see new patterns, particularly recurring words or phrases, or similar concepts which may be expressed slightly differently between data items and participants but have some commonality. This can be time-consuming, and it can be tempting to skip it, but it will be time well spent. If more than one researcher is involved, each one will need to go through this process before moving on to the next steps.

Phase 2: Creating initial codes

Once researchers have familiarised themselves with the data, the next step is to generate the initial codes. A code is the most basic building block of data analysis and identifies a feature of the data that is of interest to the researcher (Boyatzis, 1998; Braun and Clarke, 2013). The example case study 5.1 illustrates this process.

Case study 5.1: Coding interview transcripts

Emmanuel is a researcher who has been asked by a children's hospital to investigate how high-profile child deaths affect nursing staff in children's services. He interviewed a number of front-line children's nurses. Having reread his interview transcripts thoroughly, Emmanuel started coding his first transcript and began with the following passage from a children's nurse (Table 5.1).

Table 5.1 Interview transcript

Transcript		Codes
Interviewer:	*How does a high-profile child death affect you as a children's nurse?*	'A lot more anxiety'
		'Little supervision'
Participant 1:	*It creates a lot more anxiety in front-line nurses, definitely. And it's hard to deal with that anxiety when you get so little clinical supervision. So, you tend to find ways to cope with it, some positive and some negative. The positive ways are that I tend to go out of my way to document everything in the smallest detail and make sure I've got my paperwork constantly up to date. The negative ways are that this means that I work even longer hours, as I can't do all the paperwork during a normal shift, so I have to stay behind and get off late, and so I get more tired, so it's more likely I'll make a mistake.*	'Positive ways of coping' 'Negative ways of coping'

Comment

As you can see, the transcript is divided into two columns. In the first column are the words of the participants, while the second column is for Emmanuel's codes. The transcript should be double-line-spaced, and it can be helpful to number the lines for ease of reference.

Reflecting the participant's words

In the example shown in the case study, Emmanuel has decided that the best way to reflect the participant's words is to reproduce them faithfully. Technically, this is known as *emic* or 'in vivo' coding because it relates to the words and phrases used by participants. The alternative approach is *etic* or analytical codes, which are devised by the researcher and usually relate to the theoretical perspective that underpins the analysis. For example, if the same data were analysed using a psychoanalytic framework, the coding for 'ways of coping' might be termed 'defence mechanisms'.

The process of coding data involves breaking it down into its smallest parts (codes) before rebuilding it into major patterns (themes). To use a metaphor, imagine the transcript is made up of children's coloured bricks. When researchers are coding data, they are breaking down what participants have said into its smallest constituent parts (bricks) and deciding what colour each part should be. For example, participants talked about 'negative ways of coping' during the interview: each example of this can be coded and given a particular colour (e.g. red). All of the 'red bricks' (data extracts coded as red) within the interview and across all of the interviews can be gathered together.

The metaphor has its limitations because it suggests that the coloured building bricks are already contained in the data and jump out with minimal effort, whereas in reality this is a complex process that can take many iterations before the 'colours' become evident. It may be tempting to think of data analysis as being a passive process of themes 'emerging' from interview or focus group transcripts, but it needs to be a much more active and scholarly event which can take days.

'Emerging codes or themes' can, at one level, be a reassuring image because it presents the view that knowledge exists out there to be discovered and implies that data analysis is an objective, scientific process in which the analyst has an objective role. For experienced researchers this is not a sustainable view as data analysis is an active process in which choices are continually made and to which they bring their previous experience and the experience of interviewing participants. Some might regard these as 'contaminants' or 'biases' that should be removed in order to obtain an 'objective' view but, in qualitative research, removing the self and personal experiences from the research process is neither possible nor desirable. Instead, it is about being reflexive – about questioning personal assumptions and views and being open about them in data analysis and subsequent write-ups.

What is important is that equal attention is given, as material that may seem unpromising initially may become important later. Although this will rarely be discussed in research reports, a large number of codes will initially be developed, and this will allow researchers to generate potential themes while also retaining some of the surrounding data to help to understand the context. Some sections of transcripts may not be coded because there is discussion or explanation of a concept in some detail, while other sections may receive more than one code if many concepts are being outlined: *You can code individual extracts in as many different 'themes' as they fit into – so an extract may be uncoded, coded once, or coded many times, as relevant* (Braun and Clarke, 2006, page 89).

Once the transcripts are coded and there are data extracts relating to a particular code, these are grouped together with some identifying information for ease of analysis when building themes. For example, see the case study below.

Case study 5.2: Theming topics

As Emmanuel undertakes further interviews, he will add any further mention of 'negative ways of coping'. At the end of the process, he will have a file called 'negative ways of coping' that will contain all of the participants' words when they were discussing this topic (Table 5.2).

Table 5.2 Coded extracts

Code: 'negative ways of coping'
Participant 1
The negative ways are that this means that I work even longer hours, as I can't do all the paperwork during a normal shift, so I have to stay behind and get off late, and so I get more tired, so it's more likely I'll make a mistake. Line 22

> **Participant 2**
>
> *I find that a high-profile child death can have a negative effect because I tend to cope with it by going to my manager all the time for every minor decision because I feel less anxious if I share the responsibility.* Line 44
>
> **Participant 3**
>
> *I find that, after a high-profile child death, I document everything very carefully and defensively. Rather than writing your notes and thinking 'how would this look if the parents read it?', you start thinking 'how would this look if it was read by an internal investigation?' (Pause) It's quite frightening really, I try not to think about it.* Line 72

This is time-consuming when done properly but is an essential step; the raw transcripts containing thousands of words are being sifted and the building blocks of data analysis are being put together to inform and give coherent themes.

By the end of this stage, there will be a large number of codes along with their related data extracts. In the next stage, themes will be identified, which means seeing which of the 'colours' seem to link together (e.g. red bricks with pink and orange bricks). These wider groupings are called themes and there are likely to be a much smaller number of them.

Phase 3: Searching for themes

When a list of the codes has been produced, the next phase is to group them into potential themes. In this phase, the researchers' aim is to see how the codes can be grouped together into broader themes and how these themes relate to each other. Using the analogy of the coloured bricks, the transcripts have already been broken down into their constituent bricks but now the bricks are being grouped into collections of similar or compatible colours (e.g. red bricks being grouped with pink and orange bricks).

So, what are themes? Themes are broader than codes and represent a higher level of abstraction. A theme *captures something important about the data in relation to the research question and represents some level of patterned response or meaning within the data set* (Braun and Clarke, 2006, page 82). There are no rigid rules because we are dealing with the complexities of meaning, so researchers need to use their judgement. If more than one researcher is involved, they will need to resolve any disagreement by discussion until consensus is reached and their agreement is a step which adds rigour to the analysis as it demonstrates that the themes generated are not just the views of one person. This must all be done transparently and consistently. While the frequency with which a topic arises in the transcript is likely to be significant, there are no hard and fast rules. For example, a rule like: 'if the theme occurs in more than 50 per cent of the interview or focus group transcripts, it is a theme' is not helpful (Braun and Clarke, 2006), and there is an argument that qualitative researchers should avoid attempts at quantification in their data analysis.

Themes will frequently have more than one concept in them, and thus themes will be the overarching concepts while subthemes are similar or related issues. For example, Emmanuel has a theme of 'ways of coping', which has two sub-themes: negative and positive ways of coping. Themes may have a clear relationship with each other; for example, whether the themes of 'ways of coping' and 'lack of supervision' are linked with the theme of 'increased anxiety of practitioners'.

As analysis progresses, some themes may become more important, while others become peripheral. Themes become more important because they say something significant about the research question or topic. Some codes do not fit into any group and can be grouped into a theme called 'miscellaneous', possibly on a temporary basis (Braun and Clarke, 2006). Eventually researchers may find they do not use all these 'miscellaneous' codes and can discard some of them.

At the end of this phrase, researchers will have developed a number of initial or candidate themes and sub-themes that can be organised into an initial thematic map (Figure 5.1).

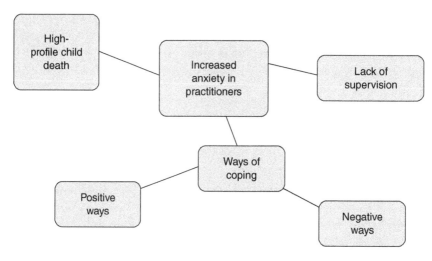

Figure 5.1   Thematic map

Phase 4: Reviewing themes

Having drawn up a list of potential or candidate themes and developed an initial thematic map, this phase focuses on reviewing and refining these themes. Data analysis, like so much of the research process, involves going back and forth between different stages in a recursive process.

In this phase, themes are reviewed at two levels. The first level is within the theme, in which all of the extracts from the transcripts are coded within that theme. As data extracts from each theme are examined, researchers will be evaluating critically whether the theme has sufficient data and whether they are sufficiently similar. If some themes have insufficient data or the data are too dissimilar then they are not sustainable themes. It may also be the case that what initially appears to be one theme needs to be split into two when the data are more carefully considered. Alternatively, your two initial themes may eventually prove to form one larger theme.

Within each theme, the data should clearly relate to it and be distinct from other themes. *Data within themes should cohere together meaningfully, while there should be clear and identifiable distinctions between themes* (Braun and Clarke, 2006, page 91).

Having reviewed codes within themes, the second level is to review across all of the transcripts. Here, researchers will review the themes overall to check that they reflect the meanings apparent in the total data set by standing back from the detailed reading of extracts to check whether the themes accurately reflect what participants said.

This all sounds easy. In fact, this is a complex but necessary step in the analysis as one frequent problem, particularly for novice researchers, is that they can end up with a lot of similar or closely related material spread across several themes, which could 'collapse down' into one major, overarching theme. This would simplify the analysis and make the write-up more convincing and coherent. Reading and rereading the themes and codes can help to overcome this; often this level of understanding develops over several days of work.

Phase 5: Defining and naming themes

Having developed a suitable thematic map, the next task is to define and refine the themes and to identify names that capture the core of what the theme is about. This requires a review of the data extracts upon which it was based. Rather than just paraphrasing the verbatim content, the key features of interest must be identified, probably in relation to your research aims and objectives or the broad area of interest. Within some themes, sub-themes are likely to be present which organise the material. These need to be named too, and these names may contribute to naming the overarching themes in which they sit.

By the end of this stage, there will be a clear idea about what is included and what is not included in each theme; this will be achieved when each theme is clear, can be described in a couple of sentences and has names that are succinct and convey a coherent sense of what the theme is about.

Phase 6: Producing the report

In research reports, each theme should receive a detailed analysis, including how it fits into the overall narrative about the data. This stage begins when researchers have decided on a final set of themes and a thematic map. Writing up will be discussed in detail in Section 4.

Qualitative data analysis software

Qualitative data analysis (QDA) software is an alternative to coding data manually. Packages such as NVivo, ATLAS.ti, MAXQDA and the Ethnograph can separate out data extracts according to the codes assigned to them and help map out how they relate to each other. These software packages can be quite expensive and are purchased by universities and by researchers as part of the grants and contracts they receive. It is necessary to have specialist training in how they work and, while in experienced hands they can be useful, the software does not actually do the analysis; it simply makes a researcher's own analysis easier as a process. See Gibbs (2018) and the websites identified at the end of the chapter for discussion of different software packages.

Focus group data analysis issues

Focus group data analysis can proceed using the same processes as the thematic analysis derived from Braun and Clarke (2006, 2013), described above. However, although this may sound obvious, the purpose of a focus group is to represent the views of a group and their analysis thus has certain considerations that are different from when individuals are being interviewed separately. Most important of these is that participants in groups interact, discuss, challenge, clarify and generally engage in a dialogue rather than simply answer questions, and this interaction needs to be considered and should be reflected in data analysis processes and in research reports. This is frequently not clear when reading research reports but is important as it can add richness by reflecting diverse viewpoints in a group and show that researchers have acknowledged this and have taken it into account rather than simply picking quotes to support their own biases. The example in the case study illustrates this.

Case study 5.3: Data from focus group discussions

Emmanuel conducted a focus group to discuss how managers at the children's hospital react to high-profile child deaths in their management practices and support of children's nurses:

> P1: *What I tend to do, is worry about it a lot in case there are any cases going on regarding children in our care which might be spotted by my nursing staff on the ward; this really gets to me when there is a high-profile case in the news as I dread something like Baby P happening here.*

Comment

This is giving only one manager's perspective, and although it is a clear example of her anxiety (which reflects what the nurses said in Emmanuel's individual interviews), it in no way reflects the views of the group. See how the picture is altered if an exchange of views is represented:

> P1: *What I tend to do, is worry about it a lot in case there are any cases going on regarding children in our care which might be spotted by my nursing staff on the ward; this really gets to me when there is a high-profile case in the news.*

P2: *I worry about it too – we all do, but let's not forget that we have invested a great deal of time and effort into establishing effective policies and procedures for safeguarding children in this directorate, and we have to have faith that these are appropriate and work as we intended.*

P3: *Look, we now have in place compulsory, yearly training for all staff on this issue. I know we can't afford to be complacent, and it would be awful if something did happen, but I do the training with them and I say it again and again, you must report anything suspicious. I give them the name and phone number of the safeguarding lead on a card so that they can phone her direct … we can't be everywhere at once as a team and we have to trust our staff to act appropriately.*

P4: *I agree but it's still a huge worry.*

P1: *Yes, you're right but I still get sleepless nights about it sometimes.*

Having included an exchange of views on the issue rather than one simple quote, it is clear now that each participant in this manager's focus group has a significant level of anxiety about issues concerning safeguarding children, but the contextual information about the Trust's response is important and helps to offset the personal anxiety as they all know that appropriate policies and procedures are in place to help staff to respond. This is a much more complex and interesting analytic point (which may be compared and contrasted, for example, between Trusts) than simply reporting the anxiety shown by Participant 1.

So, when analysing focus group data, it must be emphasised that the important subjects are not necessarily the ones that get talked about most frequently. Also, often it is when concluding questions are asked, such as 'all things considered' or 'is there anything else you'd like to add?' that participants identify the most important issues explicitly. Frequently, when the tape recording is stopped people will continue and give data that are highly relevant. Similarly, it is important to give attention to the personal context that participants use in giving their responses to the topics.

Quinn and Fantasia (2018) identify three issues concerning the use of focus group data:

1. The data derived from focus groups represent the end point of discussion within a group of people who are present at that time. They can produce rich and varied data that may not have been possible in individual interviews, as the dynamics are different. However, the dynamics can be problematic, in that people can be swayed or suppressed in their opinions by the group setting.

2. It is difficult to assess or evaluate the strength of opinion in a focus group, and even more so to try to compare this across different groups, as there is no quantitative basis for attempting such measurement. This means focus group analysis must always be tentative in this regard.

3. Attempting to make generalisations based upon focus group data is misguided; again, there is no quantitative basis for attempting generalisation. As with all qualitative research, a more important concept in relation to focus groups is that of trustworthiness, which includes credibility, transferability and confirmability.

One of the practical issues that can be challenging when transcribing focus group data is identifying which participant was speaking at any particular time. In the transcript in the case study above, each participant is given a separate number to identify them. When you are transcribing a focus group, you may find that you hear someone making a statement, but it is unclear which participant it is. This can be significant during data analysis when you are trying to establish how important particular topics are. For example, a particular topic may be mentioned three times during a focus group. It is important to establish whether the point was made by three different people or whether it is the same person making the point three times. The simplest way to address this is to ensure that you have a second person who is taking notes while you moderate the focus group, because they can take notes about the order in which people spoke and help you identify participants when the recording is unclear.

Activity 5.1 Critical thinking

Imagine that you are a student who is interested in exploring the impact on people with head injuries of moving from hospital care into residential care. You are deciding who to interview and are considering interviewing a service user, a relative, a care manager, a care assistant and a residential home manager. What problems may this raise for data analysis?

There is a brief outline answer at the end of the chapter.

Critiquing qualitative research studies

In the previous chapter, we introduced you to how to use the CASP critical appraisal tool with a qualitative paper. Question 8 on the qualitative CASP checklist is 'Was the data analysis sufficiently rigorous?' The answer to this relates to the processes we have discussed in this chapter; specifically, that appropriate processes have been followed, which are consistent with the research design and methods, and that the authors have discussed these in enough detail. If that is not the case, how can you as a reader be sure that the researchers have not simply made up their findings? For example, thinking about Braun and Clarke's six-stage model, discussed above, in order for that process to be rigorous, and be seen to be understood to be rigorous by readers, there would need to be some discussion of each of the six stages, and it's clear that the authors have not simply jumped to find themes (stage 3) without being familiar with the data (stage 1). Consider the following CASP hints:

- if there is an in-depth description of the analysis process;
- if thematic analysis is used and, if so, is it clear how the categories/themes were derived from the data?
- whether the researcher explains how the data presented were selected from the original sample to demonstrate the analysis process;

- if sufficient data are presented to support the findings;
- to what extent contradictory data are taken into account;
- whether the researcher critically examined their own role, potential bias and influence during analysis and selection of data for presentation.

Chapter summary

In this chapter, we have discussed the processes involved in analysing qualitative data and given some ideas about how to use the CASP tool to critically appraise papers that use them. Thematic analysis has been presented as a clear and systematic model for analysing qualitative data using a six-stage approach. Clarity and consistency are required in data analysis and in writing about such processes. These ideas can help inform your thinking when considering proposal writing and reading research reports that have used these techniques.

Activity: Brief outline answer

Activity 5.1   Critical thinking (pages 98)

This activity looks at problems in data analysis commentary.

Although you would gain a considerable breadth of views, it would be very difficult to develop an interview schedule and to analyse the interview data. This is because all of the participants have very different roles so it would be quite challenging to devise questions that would be relevant to all participants. It would be equally challenging to analyse participants' answers because there may be few similarities between the accounts. It could be similar to trying to write an essay in which you compare the colour red, the number seven and the country Belgium (Thurlow-Brown, 1988). It also raises ethical issues because it is very difficult to anonymise participants' comments if you have chosen people from different agencies. For example, if you interview one person from a particular agency, you may present your findings as 'the participant from the voluntary agency stated that ...'. Since there is only one participant from a voluntary agency, it is often easy for readers who are familiar with the agencies to be able to identify the staff member who is being referred to. It is more realistic to choose a smaller number of perspectives, such as service users and carers or care managers and residential staff, in order to ensure that your data can be analysed and reported in a straightforward way.

Further reading

Braun, V and Clarke, V (2006) Using thematic analysis in psychology. *Qualitative Research in Psychology*, 3: 77–101.

A classic and well-written article that covers the theoretical and pragmatic issues around thematic analysis and presents a clear and detailed account of the process.

Braun, V and Clarke, V (2013) *Successful Qualitative Research: A Practical Guide for Beginners.* London: Sage.

A good qualitative research textbook with excellent coverage of data analysis.

Clark, T, Foster, L, Bryman, A and Sloan, L (2021) *Bryman's Social Research Methods* (6th edition). Oxford: Oxford University Press.

Good discussion of qualitative analysis and an excellent all-round research textbook.

Miles, MB, Huberman, AM and Saldaña, J (2019) *Qualitative Data Analysis: A Methods Sourcebook* (4th edition). Thousand Oaks, CA: Sage.

New edition of a classic and highly influential textbook that provides a good background to qualitative data analysis.

Useful websites

https://eprints.hud.ac.uk/id/eprint/3059/

Online QDA provides a set of learning materials for those beginning to use Computer Assisted Qualitative Data Analysis (CAQDAS) packages as well as manual forms of data analysis. It is based at Huddersfield University and is closely connected to the CAQDAS Networking Project.

www.surrey.ac.uk/computer-assisted-qualitative-data-analysis

The CAQDAS Networking Project provides practical support, training and information in the use of a range of software programs designed to assist with qualitative data analysis. It is based at Surrey University and works closely with Online QDA (see above).

Chapter 6 Using and critiquing research methods: surveys and experimental designs

Chapter aims

After reading this chapter, you should be able to:

- describe the features of surveys;
- describe the features of experimental designs;
- understand the key issues of validity and reliability in surveys and in experimental designs;
- be aware of the ethical issues around experimental research;
- use your knowledge to critique studies.

Introduction

In this chapter we will look at common quantitative study designs: we will first consider features of questionnaire surveys, and then move on to experimental and quasi-experimental designs, including RCTs and related basic study designs. Issues of validity and reliability will be considered, as will sample size and power calculation. We will start from the perspective of choosing potential strategies when planning a proposal and will refer to aspects that are important when critiquing research findings.

Survey designs

Questionnaires are a popular and widely used research method, which is at least partly because we are familiar with their use in everyday life and with the underlying principle of considering information that has been obtained from a sample of people to be representative of a much larger group of people.

Questionnaires originate from the survey tradition, which has a long history in the social sciences. The terms 'questionnaire' and 'survey' are often used interchangeably. *Surveys* are a type of non-experimental study design, and are used to study large groups or populations, usually using a standardised, quantitative approach to identify beliefs, attitudes, behaviour and other characteristics. Questionnaires form a key research method for collecting survey data, but surveys can use a range of methods, such as highly structured, face-to-face or telephone interviews. Consequently, surveys are an overall research design, whereas questionnaires are one of the research tools used within surveys.

Surveys can be cross-sectional or longitudinal. A cross-sectional survey would be administered at one point in time only to assess views or attributes of a sample. Longitudinal surveys would be administered once and then again at a later date, maybe several times, to assess how the sample's views were changing or developing.

The long tradition of survey research has led to a considerable amount of rules and guidance about constructing and administering questionnaires. This chapter aims to address the key issues in questionnaire research to enable you to understand them and to consider whether they might be the most appropriate method for answering your research questions and so be useful in your proposals.

We will discuss when it is appropriate to use questionnaires compared to other research methods. A five-stage model of developing questionnaire research will be presented, from deciding on a research question and design through to analysing the data. In this process, ethical issues and sampling strategies will be explored and the strengths and limitations of questionnaires will be discussed. A case study, activities and practical tips will be provided to illustrate issues in the management of a questionnaire research project.

When is it appropriate to use questionnaires?

Questionnaires are most appropriate when straightforward quantitative information is required, from a large number of people, on a relatively well-understood topic. For a topic requiring more exploratory research using data that are complex and uncertain from a smaller number of people, qualitative research methods such as interviews and focus groups may be more appropriate.

Consider the following case study.

Case study 6.1: Choosing a design

Luciana is a final-year nursing student who is interested in coping mechanisms and resilience amongst student nurses who complete their programme. She is considering two research questions:

1. Do nursing students feel that their university could offer more counselling and support to students?
2. How stressed are students in the last year of their nursing programmes?

Activity 6.1   Decision making

Put yourself in Luciana's position. Which question do you think would be more appropriate for using questionnaires? Write a rationale for your answer.

There is a brief outline answer at the end of the chapter.

When planning to use a questionnaire, one of the most common mistakes is to include a significant number of open-ended, qualitative questions. This is problematic for two reasons. First, participants are unlikely to fill out the questionnaire completely because they do not want to keep writing long passages, so some questions will be ignored, and participants may give up part way through. Second, it can be difficult to understand the answers they give as participants may respond to a question in very different ways and there is no opportunity to clarify responses with participants, unlike other methods such as interviews and focus groups. This may result in significant amounts of missing or confusing data. Consequently, it is best to keep the number of open-ended questions to an absolute minimum (Clark et al., 2021). It is preferable to use existing valid and reliable measures that have been tested and found to be appropriate and useful in similar populations to those you want to study.

Research summary 6.1

The most famous example of using open-ended, qualitative questions inappropriately comes from Karl Marx, whose workers' survey (*enquête ouvrière*) was a questionnaire sent out to 25,000 French socialists and others. It had 101 questions, finishing with the following question:

> *What is the general, physical, intellectual, and moral condition of people employed in your trade?*
>
> (Marx and Griffiths, 2018, page 39)

Unsurprisingly, there is no record of any questionnaires being returned.

The five stages of completing a questionnaire survey

The process of completing a questionnaire survey consists of five stages:

1. deciding a research question and design;
2. searching for a questionnaire tool already in existence that has been shown to be valid and reliable or, if none exists, developing a questionnaire from scratch, including ethical issues;
3. sampling;
4. data collection;
5. data analysis.

Stage 1: Deciding a research question and design

This stage involves deciding a research question and if there is a specific hypothesis to be tested. A *hypothesis* is *a statement about the relationship between two or more variables and predicts an expected outcome* (Moule, 2020, page 38). It is a hunch coming from reading the literature, a theory or observations and experience and it must be capable of being tested (Nardi, 2018).

As questionnaires are most often and most effectively used in quantitative research, variables should be identified that are most relevant to the research question. *Variables* are attributes that can take on different values with different cases and could include your participants' attitudes, beliefs, behaviour, knowledge, or some other characteristic. We shall follow through this process with Luciana as she develops her research project.

Case study 6.2: Using questionnaires

Luciana is interested in using questionnaires to measure her fellow students' attitudes towards stress in their professional training. She wants to know how severe this might be in comparison with other students on other programmes. She is interested in whether participants' responses differ according to year of study, age, gender and family responsibilities.

In the case study, Luciana may have a hypothesis that older students will report lower levels of stress than younger students. How might she test this? If she demonstrates that her hypothesis can be supported, will it show that older students are less stressed?

If she includes questions about students' age and analyses them with data from her questionnaire, she will be able to test this hypothesis. With regard to the second question, remember that Luciana's project is a survey of the student nurses rather than an observation of their lives or exploration of their feelings. Consequently, proving her hypothesis means that older students are more likely to be less stressed than younger ones. The question of why this might be could be discussed in relation to the literature (have older people developed more robust coping strategies?). She could also compare her data with data reported for other students on other programmes. Luciana could make recommendations about how to address it, but this would not have been a central feature of her own study.

Operationalisation, validity and reliability

The process of deciding which indicators to use when measuring variables is called *operationalisation*; that is, how to convert an abstract concept into a quantifiable measure. For example, Luciana wants to measure student nurses' stress, and has chosen to use a rating scale completed by students because it is specific and measurable. She wants to see the relationship between this and the students' age, gender and family responsibilities.

Two key concepts when choosing the indicators to be measured are validity and reliability. *Validity* refers to whether what we are measuring is what we think we are measuring. *Reliability* refers to how consistent or stable a particular measure is. To use an example, imagine that Luciana wanted to measure how stressed student nurses are and decided that the best way to do this is by measuring their physical height. Since height is not a measurement of stress, this would not be a valid measure because she would not be measuring what she thinks she is measuring. However, assuming she used an ordinary tape measure, it could be a reliable measurement in the sense that she would measure students repeatedly and receive the same results. But if she used a tape measure made out of elastic, it would be neither valid nor reliable because she would receive different results at different times.

It is a difficult thing to develop questionnaires that are valid and reliable from scratch and as a general rule for project planning and proposal writing it is better to use instruments that are pre-existing and have been tested by researchers and found to be valid and reliable using the measures outlined in Table 6.1. There are numerous rating scales, covering many aspects of human experience, and a quick search of the internet or of relevant academic journals in your field should find suitable ones. It may be that your programme requires you to design a questionnaire, so check before you use existing instruments. It may be appropriate to develop a questionnaire as part of a project you are planning if there isn't one already in existence, taking into account some of the issues mentioned below. Issues of validity and reliability are addressed in Table 6.1.

Table 6.1 Establishing reliability and validity in questionnaires, instruments, and rating scales(adapted from Clark et al., 2021). More information on the terminology used in this table can be found in the Further reading section of this chapter. See Clark et al. (2021)

Reliability		
Type	**Explanation**	**Means**
Stability	Shows that a measure is unchanging over time.	Administering the test to a group once, then again later, to see if the scores are the same. Known as the test–retest method; there should be a high degree of statistical correlation between the scores.
Internal reliability	Tests whether the measures are coherent and meaningful in large item scales where there are large numbers of items or questions.	The split-half method: splits the scale in half, then measures whether responses are similar in magnitude in each half, so do those who score highly in one half do so in the other? This generates a correlation coefficient. Chronbach's alpha calculates the average of all possible correlation coefficients. An acceptable value is 0.8 (range 0–1). There is a more in-depth explanation of Chronbach's alpha here **https://stats.oarc.ucla.edu/spss/faq/ what-does-cronbachs-alpha-mean/**
Interobserver consistency or interrater reliability	Most simply understood as the extent to which two or more people would score (or rate) things.	Most easily established by making sure there is consistency between observers, possibly by training.

Validity		
Type	**Explanation**	**Means**
Face validity	Achieved by demonstrating that questions or items appear to measure the concept in question.	Asking expert opinion to judge the items.
Content validity	Measures the extent to which items in a rating scale measure all the key aspects of the concept in question.	Similar to face validity but more powerful as face validity is based on expert opinion rather than more rigorous measurement.

Validity		
Type	**Explanation**	**Means**
Concurrent validity	Comparing a criterion on which attitudes are known to differ.	Measure whether attitudes do indeed differ. For example, if a new measure of job satisfaction found that attitudes to absenteeism were the same among those who liked and disliked their jobs, doubt may be cast on the items as it is likely that those who like their jobs regard absenteeism differently from those who don't.

Reliability		
Type	**Explanation**	**Means**
Predictive validity	Comparing a criterion on which attitudes are believed will differ in the future.	How well does the new measure predict future absenteeism?
Construct validity	Seeks to establish how items in a new scale compare with what has been written from a theoretical point of view: the literature might suggest a relationship between variables, but does the new measure actually show this?	Correlations would be used as statistical tests to show how far the new measures fitted with existing ideas: if we believe that happy workers are absent less, does our measure show this?
Convergent validity	How well do different sources of data on an issue agree or disagree?	Using measures of attitudes collected through different means.

These factors will need to be acknowledged and discussion presented about how you will establish one or more of the criteria for reliability and validity in any questionnaire you plan as part of your proposal. It is not simply enough to design your own, on your own, without reference to these issues. If you still plan to use one because it meets the needs of your research question, read on for further practical issues in questionnaire design.

Stage 2: Developing a questionnaire for an undergraduate project or dissertation

The process of developing a questionnaire requires consideration of the layout, the questions to be asked and the order in which they appear on the questionnaire. It is generally recognised that having an attractive layout is important to ensure a good response rate. A poorly designed and visually unappealing questionnaire is more likely to be consigned to the wastepaper bin or deleted from the e-mail inbox, so it is worthwhile investing time in getting it right.

'How long should a questionnaire be?' is a common student question. The golden rule is that questionnaires should *include as many questions as necessary and as few as possible* (Sarantakos, 2013).

Activity 6.2   Reflection

Think about your own experiences of filling out questionnaires. What were the best and worst parts? How long were you prepared to spend on completing a questionnaire?

(Continued)

(Continued)

When thinking about issues of questionnaire length and design, it can be useful to think about what it would be like to be the participant completing it. Most participants are prepared to spend between 5 and 15 minutes to complete a questionnaire. If a questionnaire requires considerably more time, the response rate is lower and there will be more partially completed questionnaires.

As this is a reflective exercise, there is no outline answer at the end of the chapter.

Choosing questions

When thinking of questions to be included in a questionnaire, researchers may begin by generating a range of possible questions, either alone or preferably with other people who have an interest in your research topic but who are not going to be participants. Questions generated will be reviewed and those that are not relevant discarded.

Next, they will be divided into two groups: 'need to know' and 'nice to know' (Krueger and Casey, 2015). 'Need to know' questions are vital to answering the research question whereas 'nice to know' questions are ones that are simply interesting. If all the 'nice to know' questions are included, a questionnaire will be so long that it is unlikely that many participants will ever reach the end and data will not be relevant to the research question.

Questions are traditionally divided into closed and open-ended questions. Closed questions provide participants with a fixed number of responses, while open-ended questions allow participants to respond in their own words. Closed questions with a fixed number of responses produce quantitative data that are easy to analyse.

Many of the principles of developing questions are similar to those suggested for interviews and focus groups. Ensure that questions are clear and unambiguous, without confusion and vagueness. Questions containing two elements should be avoided, such as 'did you enjoy your lectures and your practice placement?' Participants may have different responses to different parts of the question, so are likely to respond to one part only. Participants provide more reliable responses to questions that relate to their own direct experience rather than more general questions that encourage speculation and generalisations. Questions that require memory recall should be realistic.

Questions should not be repetitive. It is quite common for the initial drafts of questionnaires to ask the same question in different forms, which is confusing to participants. Language that is particularly emotional or value-laden should be avoided, as should leading questions (i.e. questions that suggest a particular response). Piloting draft questionnaires is very useful. Ensure that questions are clear and free from jargon and abbreviations (e.g. 'how did your course prepare you to meet the new NMC standards?'). These are likely to antagonise participants.

Asking 'why' questions is generally discouraged in questionnaire research. 'Why' questions suggest to participants that they should provide a rational response to what might be a decision based upon impulse, habit, tradition or other non-rational processes (Krueger and Casey, 2000). If so, participants are likely to provide an intellectual rationalisation that bears little relation to the real process.

Avoid negative questions, particularly double negatives. Participants often accidently read negative questions as positive questions and answer them accordingly. Double negatives are simply confusing.

A final issue is whether you should offer a 'don't know' option. Clark et al. (2021) argue that this is problematic, particularly when you are asking a question about attitudes. Although there is a possibility that participants will choose it as an easy option, leaving it out would force participants either to select an attitude they do not hold or not answer the question at all.

Deciding question order

Different sections of the questionnaire should flow like a conversation, following a logical order, and move from the familiar to the least familiar to enable participants to begin with what they know best. More objective questions should come first and move to more subjective questions as participants become more comfortable. Sensitive questions should be left to later in the questionnaire, but not at the end. As participants can become tired, have fairly straightforward questions at the end, such as participants' age, gender and ethnicity.

One technique that can aid the development of rating scales is factor analysis. This is a complex technique and in writing a proposal you would not be expected to get to grips with it, but it is common to see studies in academic journals using factor analysis. It is used to refine rating scales where there are many items (questions) by a procedure, which indicates where these items tend to group together in clusters (factors) of similar ideas. This could indicate that the items in the scale have an inherent structure. So, for example, in a draft scale with 100 questions these might fall into four factors each containing 15 items (60 items in total). The remaining 40 may be barely relevant and could be discarded. Thus, a potentially 100-item-long questionnaire or rating scale would be reduced to a smaller 60. The four factors would be given names relating to their content, which would add structure and also indicate key theoretical aspects of the concepts being studied (Clark et al., 2021).

Choosing the format for responses

You can choose a number of different formats for how you want participants to respond. Whichever response format is used, it is essential to give clear instructions to participants about how questions should be answered:

- Exact responses: these require a specific answer (e.g. the number of pre-qualifying years of social work experience).
- Category responses: these require participants to select one response from a list of categories (e.g. pre-qualifying experience expressed as 0–2 years, 3–4 years).
- Dichotomous responses: these are usually in the form of yes/no answers but could be other dichotomous responses (e.g. male/female).
- Likert-scale questions: these usually require participants to select a response along a sliding scale of agreement. The most common format for a Likert scale is to have two extreme positions divided by a five-point scale, though a seven-point scale can be used to distinguish subtle gradations.
- Semantic differential scale: two opposite adjectives are placed on a numerical scale and participants choose which number best represents their view.
- Graphic scales: graphic representations, such as faces or ladders, are used to represent participants' attitudes. These are commonly used in learning disability research and can be particularly helpful with children. Visual analogue scales (VASs) are also popular in, for example, pain assessment. Patients may be asked to rate their pain from 0 to 100, with 100 being the most severe ever. After the administration of analgesia, if the patient were asked to re-rate the pain, the effectiveness of the analgesia could be assessed.
- Constant-sum scales and pie charts: participants are asked to score two or more alternatives so that the scores add up to a fixed amount or are presented with a blank pie chart and asked to divide it up to represent the relative importance of particular elements.

A key factor in determining what format you wish to use is how you are going to analyse the data afterwards. Consequently, it is worthwhile reading this section alongside Chapter 7, which describes some of the statistical tests that you can use with your data and some of the limitations of particular types of data. If data analysis is not planned, there is a danger that the data will be collected in a form that does not allow the use of statistical procedures required.

Ethical issues

There are ethical issues to be addressed when using questionnaires, though questionnaires are generally regarded as having lower ethical risks than more intrusive research methods. Unlike interviews and focus groups, questionnaires offer the possibility of anonymity because the researcher may not know the identity of participants, which is a higher level of protection than confidentiality. This makes questionnaires useful for researching sensitive topics because participants are more likely to disclose sensitive material if they can remain anonymous. Promising anonymity is problematic if questionnaires are returned via e-mail as the researcher will usually be able to identify participants, but you will always be able to offer confidentiality. However, online survey programs such as SurveyMonkey allow the researcher to make responses completely anonymous as the software can be set to collect no identifying information, not even the IP address of the computer used to complete it. Such survey programs are easy to use, will do some data analysis for you, and allow you to e-mail or embed your survey in a webpage or social media feed like X (formerly Twitter). This makes administration much simpler and easier than photocopying paper items, and allows wide, even international distribution.

Since the GDPR legislation was introduced in 2018, it is no longer enough to assume that consent to use the data has been given implicitly by completing and returning the questionnaire in whatever format. Consent must be explicitly spelled out, including issues of confidentiality and anonymity, right to withdraw data and protection from harm, and so participants require information about the research, which is normally contained in information sheets or covering letters. Also, if the survey will be entirely anonymous, it must be made clear that it will not be possible to withdraw data as there is no way of identifying from whom it originated. You may have to go through the Health Research Authority and local NHS Trust research governance processes and a university ethics committee for approval prior to commencing the research unless you plan to recruit only via social media.

Stage 3: Sampling

The next stage is deciding how you are going to select the sample. *Sampling* refers to the process of selecting the participants who will be involved in the study. The sample of participants is chosen from the total possible group of people, known as the *population.*

The two main types of sampling are probability and non-probability sampling.

Probability or *random sampling* uses mathematical techniques based upon probability theory to select research participants who are representative of the overall population. It is the most common sampling approach used in questionnaire research and random sampling increases the likelihood that the results will be generalisable to a wider population. Non-probability sampling is a weaker form of sampling but is still used in many studies for convenience (hence convenience sampling).

Samples can be divided up (or stratified) in certain ways, such as age, gender and ethnicity, although this may not be necessary, particularly if the resultant sample size is relatively small. For example, having one or two people from a specific ethnic group is too small a sample size to be able to make any worthwhile generalisations. In research, it is always wise to be realistic about what can be claimed based upon evidence and it is better to understate rather than overstate a case.

Choosing the sample is important, as it will influence the data received. A famous example is the *Chicago Daily Tribune* erroneously announcing that Republican Thomas Dewey had won the US presidential election in 1948, rather than Democrat Harry Truman. This occurred because the newspaper had seen polls that predicted a Dewey victory, but the poll had been conducted using a biased sample. The polls were conducted using fixed quotas from rural and urban populations that had not been updated to reflect the recent move from rural areas into cities. Consequently, they underrepresented urban voters who were more likely to vote for Democrat Truman.

Clark et al. (2021) identify four main types of probability sampling: *simple random sampling, systematic sampling, stratified random sampling and multi-stage cluster sampling.*

Simple random sampling

This is the most basic form of random sampling, in which cases are selected randomly using random number tables or an online random generator (such as **www.randomizer. org**). Each unit of the population has an equal chance of being included in the sample and this method eliminates human bias. However, it is only possible if you have a list of all people in your population (i.e. a sampling frame).

Systematic sampling

This is a variation of the simple random sample, in which cases are selected in a systematic way (e.g. choosing every tenth case). It is important to ensure the sampling frame (list of potential participants) is not structured in a way that would make it non-random and, if so, to randomise the order of the list.

Stratified random sampling

If there are particular factors to be concentrated upon, the sample can be made to ensure sufficient representation. In the case study, Luciana may be interested in whether gender makes a difference in students' attitudes about their stress levels. She could establish the overall gender proportions in the nursing student group and choose a proportionate sample for each gender. Having established the overall target number of participants for each gender, she would then choose specific participants using simple random sampling or systematic sampling.

Multi-stage cluster sampling

When a sample is geographically spread, cluster sampling enables the grouping together of potential participants. Imagine that Luciana wanted to research nursing students across the UK. It would be unrealistic to sample randomly every student, as that would need students from every university. Instead, cluster sampling would enable her to choose a smaller number of universities through random sampling. She may wish to group the universities further (e.g. choosing regions) and randomly select them within specific regions (Clark et al., 2021).

One potential problem with recruitment via social media is that it is unlikely that you will be able to target segments or strata of a population in the same way as the methods described above. You will be able to build demographic questions into your questionnaire, as well as other variables, and X/Tweet or Facebook relevant sites that represent particular elements or interests, but that may not be as accurate as other methods.

Stage 4: Data collection

Having developed a questionnaire, it is important to pilot it because, unlike interviews or focus groups, there is no opportunity to explain ambiguous or unclear questions. Questions that make sense to the authors may not make sense to participants, who may consistently misread questions, so such questions need to be reworded.

One aim is to maximise your response rate. Having developed a clear and attractive questionnaire, the response rate can be improved by using follow-up letters with additional copies of the questionnaire. This can be fruitful but should not delay a project too much. A general rule of thumb is that about three-quarters of completed questionnaires should be returned in the first three weeks. The final quarter may respond to a reminder letter, but there will come a point when the project must proceed to the next stage. Distributing questionnaires by e-mail or social media makes the whole process of administering them and sending reminders much easier and cheaper, however digital methods are variable in their effectiveness: some studies indicate a higher response rate than other methods, while other studies argue that response rates are lower than face-to-face methods; it is also possible to get the format of a digital survey quite wrong and inhibit completion (Williamson et al., 2018). Many of the survey software packages now allow upload of e-mails and will distribute the surveys for you, rather than you having to construct an e-mail list yourself.

Stage 5: Analysing your data and presenting your findings

The analysis of your data using descriptive statistics will be discussed in detail in Chapter 7. It would be worthwhile reading this now to understand how data collection progresses to analysis.

Strengths and limitations of questionnaires

Questionnaires have a number of strengths and weaknesses.

Their strengths are as follows:

- Questionnaires are relatively inexpensive and quick to administer.
- Participants can respond when it is convenient for them and there is a greater assurance of anonymity.
- There are fewer opportunities for errors or bias caused by the presence of the interviewer. For example, participants may give answers that are sociably acceptable but not accurate (social desirability bias).

- The questions are asked in a stable and consistent manner, with no interviewer variability. They allow greater coverage because participants can be approached more easily and there are no problems around 'non-contacts', where participants are not available at the time.

Their weaknesses are as follows:

- Questionnaires do not allow opportunities for probing and clarifying responses with participants, or for collecting additional information (e.g. observation) while the questionnaire is being completed.
- The researcher does not have an opportunity to motivate the participant to complete all of the questions or ensure the questions are answered in the correct order, if relevant.
- There are limitations as to how long participants are willing to spend on completing a questionnaire.
- Only a very limited number of open questions can be asked, because participants do not want to write large amounts.
- They are less appropriate for people with literacy difficulties or for whom English is not a first language.
- The identity of the participant is not known, so the researcher cannot be sure the right person has completed the questionnaire.
- Non-response or a low response rate hinders the analysis and interpretation of results.

Critiquing survey designs

Numerous tools exist for critiquing survey designs but unfortunately CASP does not provide one. The one from the Centre for Evidence Based Management (CEBM) is available in full here **https://cebma.org/resources/tools/critical-appraisal-question naires/** and asks a series of questions related to the issues we have discussed above, including sample size and representativeness of the population, response rate, validity and reliability of the instruments (questionnaires) used, statistical significance and confidence intervals, and the applicability of the results to your own organisation. You can use this CEBM critical appraisal tool in exactly the same way as you would any others. Read your survey paper, make notes about the issues that the CEBM tool raises and then read around those issues using relevant literature to construct an argument about the strengths and/or limitations of your chosen paper.

Experimental designs

An experimental approach involves setting up a research study in which the outcome is not known (Donnan, 2015). The intention is to compare the effects of some new treatment or procedure administered to one group of patients with those in another group receiving either 'normal care' or a placebo (and so do not experience anything novel). The study is designed to test researchers' hypotheses, or research questions, about the effectiveness of the new treatment. The RCT is often described as the gold standard in this type of research; this approach is able to indicate as closely as possible whether or not hypotheses are correct when conducted in a rigorous fashion (although the accuracy of this term is disputed by, for example, Cartwright (2007)). If there was no control or comparison group, it is possible that participants might gain benefit just because something new is being done to them; the mind can produce all kinds of physical and psychological responses to treatments and placebos. The Hawthorne effect occurs when an effect noted in a research study could occur because participants know they are involved in the study (Moule, 2020). Thus, a control group is needed to assess whether the new treatment works over and above any possible Hawthorne effect.

Essential features of an RCT

For a study to be a true experiment, the following features apply (Donnan, 2015; Tilling et al., 2005; Williamson et al., 2010b).

Comparison and control groups

These are required to test a hypothesis: variables will be manipulated, and outcomes assessed between the experimental and control group(s). In this way, extraneous variables are controlled out (external influences are removed so that researchers can be sure that the effects noted are due to the actions of the intervention and not some other factors) and internal validity is high.

Sampling

As it is not possible to include all potentially eligible subjects of a population, samples must be taken, and these should theoretically be random samples. However, practical considerations mean that researchers often use convenience samples. Other sampling methods include cluster sampling, where groups of sites such as GP practices or hospitals would be included, and stratified random sampling, where sampling takes place to reflect some characteristic in a population, such as age or sex.

Sample size and power calculations

Researchers should plan the number of participants to be recruited based on upfront calculations rather than guesswork. In a proposal you would need to demonstrate that you were aware of the importance of having the correct sample size and write about how this could be demonstrated. Having too many participants in the study exposes people to unnecessary risk and gives the researcher an unnecessary recruitment burden: why have 1,000 people in a study when 200 (100 in each arm of a trial) would be sufficient? Having too few runs the risk of missing statistically significant findings (type II errors). In planning a proposal as part of an undergraduate piece of work you would be unlikely to be expected to do sample size estimation and power calculations but would be expected to write coherently about what they mean and why they are important. As the Consolidated Standards of Reporting Trials (CONSORT) statement puts it:

> *The sample size for a trial needs to be planned carefully, with a balance between medical and statistical considerations. Ideally, a study should be large enough to have a high probability (power) of detecting as statistically significant a clinically important difference of a given size if such a difference exists. The size of effect deemed important is inversely related to the sample size necessary to detect it; that is, large samples are necessary to detect small differences.*

(Moher et al., 2010, page 8)

What this means is that researchers, in advance, should work out the numbers they require and the effect size that these numbers will be able to detect. This will typically be expressed in a short paragraph saying they calculated that (say) 100 participants were required in each group to detect a clinically significant effect with a power of, for example, 0.8 at an α level of 0.05 (α corresponds to the p value and indicates the acceptable risk of chance findings or type I errors, set by convention at 0.05 or 5 per cent – more on this in Chapter 7); 0.8 power (or 80 per cent) indicates the power that the study has to determine the effect size. The desired level of chance in the clinical results will be dependent on what is under study, and researchers will determine what a large or small effect size is relative to their study and existing literature. For example, Powell et al. (2001) wanted to work out what a clinically significant difference might be on a VAS for measuring pain in children. On a scale which measured 100 mm, they found that the smallest clinically significant difference was 10 mm, meaning that patients could feel that level of difference if their pain was getting better or worsening. Any RCT examining analgesia regimes in children should therefore have large enough numbers of participants to determine this minimum clinically significant difference (10/100 mm) and researchers would need to work out in advance what the number of participants would be to be able to measure this 10 mm difference; the study would need a certain number to be adequately powered (the power to detect 10/100 mm change on the VAS). If they recruited less, it would be underpowered. Researchers might take the view that they want to be able to measure only 1 mm difference for some reason. This is much less than we know to be necessary to show clinical significance on this VAS, and in that case the numbers in the study would need to be substantially higher than if they only aim to be able to measure the 10 mm difference. To gain the precision to detect relatively small changes, relatively large samples will be required.

Eligibility of subject

Clear protocols should indicate inclusion and exclusion criteria (such as age and sex) for participants, to ensure that those enrolled in the study are appropriate and the sample is relatively homogeneous.

Fully informed consent

One key aspect of the practicalities of undertaking an RCT is the extent to which informed consent can be gained; without informed consent the study would be unethical. So, even though there may be a risk of harm to the patients in some new treatment, or less beneficial outcomes if they are in the placebo group, if this is explained and patients still consent then these risks are acceptable.

Randomisation

Once the sample has been chosen, is it practically and/or ethically possible to randomise participants between groups? Researchers randomly split participants between one or more study groups to avoid accidental or intentional biases in the different study groups. The groups will then be compared, and their characteristics assessed to make sure there are no biases in the group allocations. For example, if we were testing a new treatment for high blood pressure (hypertension) we would want to make sure that the mean (average) blood pressure at the start of the study in each group was similar: if our intervention group had a much lower mean blood pressure before starting the new treatment compared to the group continuing to take their existing treatment, then this would be reflected in the study findings. An element of accidental bias would have been introduced at the sampling stage and the findings would show that those in the treatment group had a lower blood pressure than the others. Similarly, randomisation of patients into different groups prevents the researchers from introducing intentional biases, which may show their study in a more favourable light if they hand-picked the 'best' participants. Methods of randomisation include simple randomisation, where random numbers are generated to allocate participants between groups; block randomisation, where participants are allocated a block and these are then split between treatment and control, to ensure that numbers allocated to each group are similar; and stratified randomisation, to ensure that characteristics such as age and sex are allocated evenly between groups.

Blinding of treatment

It should be impossible for patients, staff and researchers to know who is receiving the new treatment and who is not. This is known as double-blinding and is to avoid intentional and unintentional biases being introduced to findings if participants were treated differently because of the group they were in, or responded differently to treatment because of their own perceptions of how they were being treated. If double-blinding is not possible, a study may go ahead but it must be acknowledged that these potential biases may exist and overestimate the effects of treatment.

Analysis of differences between research or control groups

Using appropriate statistical tests and software (a common package is SPSS, the Statistical Package for the Social Sciences), statistical significance is indicated by the use of p values and/or confidence intervals (CIs) and indicates the generalisabilty of the study findings by assessing how far the results from the study sample might relate to the larger population. This will be discussed more fully in Chapter 7 on data analysis.

Limitations of RCTs

Although they may be the gold standard, even RCTs have their weaknesses and some of these are outlined below (Donnan, 2000; Tilling et al., 2005; Williamson et al., 2010b):

- Non-compliance: if participants do not routinely comply with the new treatment regime it is likely that the effects will be understated.
- Drop-out rates: if patients do not complete the study, then their data will be lost, and outcomes will not be fully assessed. This may be because of side effects of the new treatment, voluntary withdrawal or death. This can be avoided by using intention-to-treat analysis, which means that all patients who began the study are included and gives a pragmatic estimate of the effects of treatment policy rather than the actual outcomes of the study. (For a fuller explanation of this concept, see Hollis and Campbell (1999).)
- Statistical significance may be established, but are the results clinically important and can they be applied in the real world (are they clinically effective)? It is not a flaw if a study reports no statistically significant differences between active and control groups in an RCT, provided the study has been correctly conducted and is adequately powered. It may be as clinically useful to know that a new treatment or procedure does not work as it is to know that it does.
- RCTs tell us nothing on their own about the patient's experience, and sometimes 'nested qualitative studies' may be included in RCTs to gain this type of information.

There are many different types of experimental designs, and these are noted in Table 6.2. A trial would be called a quasi-experimental design if some feature such as randomisation or group concealment (double-blinding) was not possible. A quasi-experiment would also be possible if there were naturally occurring groups, such as patients already receiving some treatment. In this case, researchers would not be manipulating variables, but would be choosing the timing and extent of measurement that takes place (Punch, 2014). As a result, these would be less robust designs as if, for example, patients and staff could easily identify which group they were in (double-blinding was absent) they might be able consciously or unconsciously to influence outcomes.

Table 6.2   Randomised and non-randomised experimental designs (adapted from Tilling et al., 2005)

Design	Key features	Advantages	Disadvantages
Randomised controlled trial	Participants randomly allocated to intervention or control arm (can be placebo or 'usual treatment').	Groups balanced in everything except treatment received. If randomisation concealed, can prevent selection bias and undue potential influence from researchers.	Time and effort required to make the study robust and to implement it effectively.
Cluster randomised controlled trial	Groups of participants (e.g. GP practices or clusters of hospital Trusts in different areas) randomised to intervention or control.	Logistically easier and more suitable for some interventions (e.g. community education programmes).	Need larger sample size than individually randomised trials.
Controlled trial	Participants non-randomly assigned to intervention or control arm.	Easier to carry out than a randomised trial, as no need to prepare and conceal randomised allocation schedule.	Allocation schedule cannot be concealed, so selection bias may occur.
Before/after comparison	Data collected before and after an intervention on a group of participants, and a paired comparison made.	Reduces variability by using paired data.	Changes other than the experimental intervention may occur over the time period.
Randomised crossover trial	As above, but each participant receives control and intervention treatment in random order. Paired comparison made.	Reduces variability by using paired data.	Unsuitable for interventions with long-term effects, or conditions that change over time.
Historical	Data collected after an intervention and compared to data collected on some other group which did not experience the intervention. Unpaired comparison made.	Requires minimal data.	There may be differences between the intervention arm and the historical controls other than the experimental intervention.

Planning for analysis

As well as discussion of the key features above, a project plan for an RCT would need to contain specific information on how the numerical data were to be analysed, including what variables were to be assessed and what statistical tests would be used to test for differences between the intervention and the control group. Issues of sampling and data analysis contribute to the external validity of experimental designs and the generalisability of findings from the sample to the wider population. In a large measure this is their 'point': to show whether or not findings in the sample are likely to apply to all others with the condition.

A proposal should include a diagram showing the key stages, and with the stages clearly outlined. This allows readers to assess its replicability (Clark et al., 2021). The CONSORT statement (Moher et al., 2010; and see the CONSORT website: **www.consort-statement.org/home**) provides an excellent example of how the study should be mapped out, with key stages (Moher et al., 2010) presented in Figure 6.1.

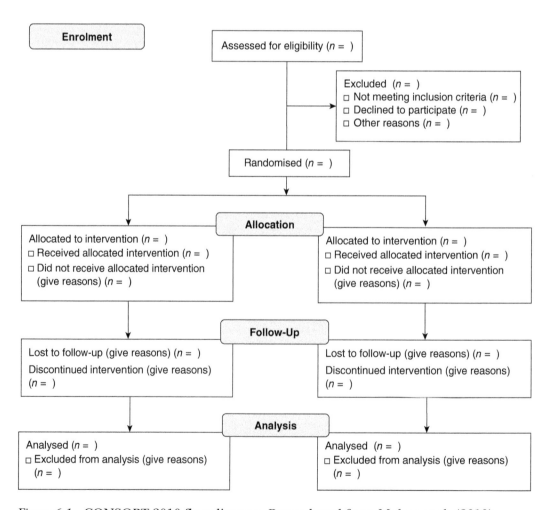

Figure 6.1 CONSORT 2010 flow diagram. Reproduced from Moher et al. (2010)

In proposals, as no actual participants have been recruited, only the stages of enrolment and allocation can be completed as there will be no follow-up or analysis, as shown in Box 6.1 (adapted from Moher et al., 2010).

Box 6.1: Enrolment and allocation for proposals

1. Numbers of eligible subjects:

   (a) excluded ($n =$)
   (b) meets/does not meet inclusion criteria ($n =$)
   (c) declined to take part ($n =$)
   (d) other reasons ($n =$)

2. Randomised between groups ($n =$)
3. Allocation:

   (a) allocated to intervention or control groups ($n =$)
   (b) received intervention or control ($n =$)
   (c) did not receive intervention or control (reasons) ($n =$)

It is imperative that researchers writing proposals for RCTs access this CONSORT website as it is an internationally recognised consensus on planning and reporting RCTs with lots of valuable resources.

Ethical issues

In proposals, there needs to be more depth about ethical issues. We have outlined key concerns of RCTs above in terms of the need for informed consent and of exposing participants to risks associated with introducing or withholding new treatments or interventions, and these would need to be more fully discussed in a proposal. One thing to consider about potential risks in RCTs from an ethical point of view is that there must be sufficient uncertainty about whether the intervention works or not to allow the trial to go ahead. If it is certain that the intervention is better than usual care a study should not proceed (Tilling et al., 2005) as there is no scientific justification for it: we already know that the intervention works best and giving another group lesser treatment is unethical. Similarly, use of placebos can be unethical and so new interventions are usually compared with 'usual care'. For example, in a study testing some new analgesic regime postsurgery, it would be unethical to trial this against a placebo as it is already well established that effective analgesic regimes exist and to expose patients to surgery without suitable postoperative pain relief would be very unpleasant for them.

However, it is important that researchers are allowed to investigate areas where there is genuine debate about clinical care. It seems axiomatic for nurses and midwives that adrenalin ought to be given in cardiac arrest situations; it is in the UK Resuscitation

Guidelines after all. Concern about whether or not giving adrenalin (epinephrine) caused more serious neurological complications in out-of-hospital cardiac arrest led to a clinical trial called Paramedic 2 (University of Warwick, see **https://warwick. ac.uk/fac/sci/med/research/ctu/trials/critical/paramedic2**), in which cardiac arrest patients were randomised to receive either epinephrine or a placebo by attending paramedics, in a double-blinded placebo-controlled RCT. How is this ethical? Because there is genuine scientific debate about use of this medication in out-of-hospital cardiac arrest. Potential participants were unconscious or near to it and could not consent, but there was a mechanism for opting out of the study in advance, rather than consenting to be included. This study gained ethical approval despite these ethical dilemmas because of the overriding scientific importance of the area. Perkins et al. (2018) reported the findings, which are that patients given epinephrine were more likely to survive and, whilst there was no statistically significant difference in positive neurological outcomes between placebo and epinephrine groups at the time of hospital discharge, severe neurologic impairment was present in more of the survivors in the epinephrine group than in the placebo group (39 of 126 patients [31.0 per cent] vs 16 of 90 patients [17.8 per cent]). This is an important result: more people survive with adrenalin, but they are likely to be in a worse neurological state. It warrants further investigation in regard to changing practice; it is after all only one study, but it is a vindication of the decision to go ahead with the trial.

Other particular ethical concerns in RCTs include the vulnerability of participants. Coercion in all forms should be avoided. The relationship between clinical staff and sick people makes them more vulnerable than healthy adults, and this must be mitigated and discussed in proposals. Written consent is essential, so a written participant information sheet (PIS) and a consent form are required, and these should be included as appendices in proposals. Ethical clearance will be required from the Health Research Authority, as will IRAS capacity and capability approval and, for students, approval from the university committee.

Critiquing RCTs

CASP has a tool for critically appraising RCTs, and students should use that in the same way that they have used CASP tools previously.

> Question 2: Was the assignment of patients to treatments randomised?

Hints

- how this was carried out;
- was the allocation sequence concealed from researchers and patients?

Although randomisation of participants between groups is the gold standard for RCTs, what if we cannot randomise? What if we can only represent pre-existing groups for some reason, like, for example, clinical need or diagnosis? Imagine we are interested in pain and analgesia post-breast surgery for different procedures. We could not randomise women to have a lumpectomy (a minimally invasive technique that preserves breast tissues) or a more radical mastectomy; the diagnosis would determine the treatment arm. We could still manipulate the type of analgesic given and compare outcomes, but we cannot randomise this, so this would be a quasi-experimental design, which is a weaker design but the only possible way of doing this study.

> Question 4: Were patients, health workers and study personnel 'blind' to treatment?

This one gives no 'Hints' but, as we have discussed above, the issue of blinding or lack of it can cause potential bias in an RCT: if researchers, clinical staff and patients know that participants are in a particular research group, and having something that might be good for them, they might alter their behaviour or responses to treatment in subtle ways. Thus, double-blinding is the gold standard, but single-blinding might be the only possible, pragmatic way of conducting a study: for example, if we wanted to study the impact of a new type of hospital mattress on pressure ulcer formation in hospitals it would be impossible to blind patients or staff to the type of mattress a patient was on. It would be possible for the researchers interpreting the data to be blinded, and this would then become a single-blinded study. This is a weaker design than an RCT but the only possible way of doing the study.

You will find other tools for critically appriasing RCTs in the Joanna Briggs Institute website **https://jbi.global/critical-appraisal-tools** and these have the advantage of extensive explanations of key concepts.

Observational quantitative research designs: cohort and case-control studies

In the discussions above we have talked about surveys (non-experimental study designs where variables are not manipulated) and experimental designs such as RCTs (where patients are randomised between groups, and some variables manipulated to assess differences between groups at the study end point). There is another category of study design known as observational designs; these are also non-experimental quantitative designs. 'Observational' in this context is not the same terminology as used in an ethnographical study where a person might be a participant observer. In regard to observational quantitative research designs, 'observational' means we are seeing what is occurring in naturally formed groups (cohorts) in a population, such as smokers and non-smokers: we will not be able to make people smoke cigarettes, but we need to know the consequences for people who do so. Such designs are frequently investigating epidemiological and public health issues.

One of the most famous and influential studies in UK public health was by Doll and Hill (1954) who looked at rates of lung cancer by comparing doctors who smoked with doctors who did not. This had the advantage of being research on people with a similar social class and income but was non-experimental in the sense that participants were not randomised, and no new intervention was introduced; it was observational – they were observing what happened to smokers compared with non-smokers. These results have been followed up and confirmed in many studies subsequently and have been instrumental in changing attitudes, banning advertising and increasing taxation of tobacco, as well as in the identification of quitting as the single most important public health measure an individual can take.

Case-control studies

A case-control study compares patients with a disease versus patients who do not have the disease. This is so that their past exposure to suspected aetiological factors is compared with that of controls who do not have the disease (BMJ, 2018). Case-control studies are retrospective; they look back in time (observe retrospectively) at what has happened.

An example of this might be to investigate the link between cigarette smoking and chronic obstructive pulmonary disease (COPD). The 'case' is the patient with COPD. The 'control' is the patient without COPD. Let's say that, of those with COPD most had smoked, and of those without COPD most had not (this is simplistic but a reasonable example). We want to know, so that we can make recommendations regarding public health, how much greater the odds of getting COPD are for the smokers compared with the non-smokers, and these cases (with COPD) have been matched to controls (without COPD) for confounding variables like income, age, gender and so on. This is assessed by using odds ratios (ORs), which is a type of calculation that shows, in this example, what the odds of getting COPD are if you regularly smoked cigarettes. We discuss statistical significance, how to calculate odds ratios and confidence intervals in more detail in Chapter 7. In study results you will see the odds ratio expressed as a number, so if we calculate the odds ratio for smoking and having developed COPD and find that it is 5 that means that the odds of smokers having contracted COPD were 5 times greater than non-smokers. ORs will be reported alongside the *p* value and the confidence intervals.

Cohort studies

Cohort studies can be retrospective (looking backwards) or prospective (looking forward) but are usually prospective. People are recruited to the study because of some feature like their occupation, geography or income, not because of their disease or illness status, so that the researchers can assess how likely it is that an exposure or variety of exposures causes a disease (Crandon, 2017). A cohort is a group of people who share a characteristic, such as a birthday: the whole of a cohort, or at least a subsection of a large cohort like all the people born in the UK on a particular day, might be enrolled into a cohort study and followed up for a long period of time to see if they contract illnesses or diseases and to ascertain what the causes might be.

One example is the Avon Longitudinal Study of Parents and Children (ALSPAC; Fraser et al., 2013), which was established to understand how genetic and environmental characteristics influence health and development in parents and children. All pregnant women resident in Avon who were expected to deliver their baby between 1 April 1991 and 31 December 1992 were eligible to be enrolled in the study, and 13,761 women (contributing 13,867 pregnancies) were recruited. These women have been followed over the last 19–22 years. The research team has examined a range of measures, looking to see what illnesses these mothers and their children might have suffered and if they can identify why. The team has produced numerous academic publications. One example is that from O'Connor et al. (2002) where they examined the association between maternal antenatal anxiety and children's emotional problems at 4 years. They found that anxious mothers did indeed have more anxious children at 4 years, and theorised that this might be because maternal mood can influence brain development in the womb. Boys and girls were both approximately twice as anxious (OR 2.14 and 1.88, respectively) if their mothers were anxious (defined by clinical assessments). Although this study reports odds ratios, other studies may report risk ratios, which are a way of assessing the relative risk of contracting a disease or illness based on the population at risk. Odds and risk ratios are similar but not the same. We talk more about this in Chapter 7.

Critiquing case-control and cohort studies

CASP has tools for both of these observational designs. They ask questions about recruitment, exposures, confounding factors, and treatment effects, follow up and applicability. Students should use the checklists in the same way as recommended previously, which is to read your paper, make notes about the issues that the CASP tools raise and then read around those issues using the relevant literature to construct an argument about the strengths and/or limitations of your chosen paper.

Activity 6.3   Critical thinking

From Table 6.2, decide which types of study are fully experimental and which are quasi-experimental designs.

There is a brief outline answer at the end of the chapter.

Chapter summary

In this chapter, we have learnt about common quantitative study designs, surveys and experimental designs, non-experimental observational designs, and questionnaires as a research method within the survey tradition. You have been invited to consider which

(Continued)

(Continued)

types of research question are appropriate to be addressed using questionnaires. A five-stage model of developing questionnaire research has been presented, taking you from deciding your research question and design through to analysing the data you have collected. We then moved on to discuss aspects of experimental designs, particularly their strengths and weaknesses. Case-control and cohort studies were also introduced. Ethical issues and sampling strategies were explored. A case study, activities and practical tips were provided in relation to questionnaires, and, for experimental designs, process issues were outlined, and the CONSORT website strongly recommended for further information.

Activities: Brief outline answers

Activity 6.1   Decision making (page 103)

The first question is more suited to qualitative methods, such as interviews and focus groups, which can provide opportunities for participants to draw upon their experiences and reflect upon their feelings. The second question can be answered by quantitative data that measure participants' attitudes and beliefs, using valid and reliable measures that are already in existence, such as those discussed in the systematic review by Pulido-Martos et al. (2012).

Activity 6.3   Critical thinking (page 125)

From Table 6.2, decide which types of study are fully experimental and which are quasi-experimental designs:

- Fully experimental: RCT, cluster RCT, randomised crossover trial.
  - Explanation: all these have full randomisation, with concealment of group membership.
- Quasi-experimental: controlled trial, before/after comparison, historical.
  - Explanation: these do not have randomisation, or a control group.

Further reading

Bowling, A (2023) *Research Methods in Health: Investigating Health and Health Services* (5th edition). Maidenhead: Open University Press.

Bowling, A and Ebrahim, S (2005) *Handbook of Research Methods in Health: Investigation, Measurement and Analysis.* Maidenhead: Open University Press.

Both of these texts are good and informative about aspects of experimental and survey designs.

Clark, T, Foster, L, Bryman, A and Sloan, L (2021) *Bryman's Social Research Methods* (6th edition). Oxford: Oxford University Press.

This is a comprehensive research methods' textbook and contains further information about the statistical elements of this chapter.

De Vaus, DA (2014) *Surveys in Social Research* (6th edition). Abingdon, Oxon: Routledge.

Sixth edition of a classic text on survey research. Readable and authoritative.

Hollis, S and Campbell, F (1999) What is meant by intention to treat analysis? Survey of published randomised controlled trials. *British Medical Journal,* 319 (7211): 670–4.

Jadad, AR and Enkin, MW (2007) *Randomized Controlled Trials: Questions, Answers and Musings.* Oxford: Blackwell Publishing.

A good chapter on ethics and controlled trials.

Nezu, AM and Nezu, M (2008) *Evidence-Based Outcome Research: A Practical Guide to Conducting Randomized Controlled Trials for Psychosocial Interventions.* Oxford: Oxford University Press.

More advanced text with emphasis on psychological usage of controlled trials.

Sapsford, R (2007) *Survey Research* (2nd edition). London: Sage.

Useful and readable text that covers the key issues in survey research.

Torgerson, DJ and Togerson, CJ (2008) *Designing Randomised Trials in Health, Education, and the Social Sciences.* Basingstoke: Palgrave Macmillan.

Detailed text but useful for those looking for a more advanced text.

Useful websites

http://news.bbc.co.uk/1/hi/england/london/4807042.stm

BBC News website with information about a drug trial at Northwick Park Hospital that went wrong.

www.students4bestevidence.net

Students 4 Best Evidence. A network for students interested in evidence-based healthcare.

http://data-archive.ac.uk/about/projects/sqb

The Survey Question Bank is part of the Survey Resources Network, an Economic and Social Research Council (ESRC) initiative coordinated by the UK Data Archive (UKDA) at the University of Essex.

www.controlled-trials.com

Information about current controlled trials.

http://en.wikipedia.org

We would normally not recommend Wikipedia as an academic source and definitely do not recommend you quote it in assignments, but it has an excellent page on clinical trials, particularly the stages that new products go through before they get to market. Google 'clinical trials' and click on the Wikipedia source, or search for clinical trials in the Wikipedia site.

https://jbi.global/critical-appraisal-tools

JBI has a wide range of tools for critically appraising evidence.

Chapter 7 Analysing quantitative data and understanding basic statistics

Chapter aims

After reading this chapter, you should be able to:

- understand the basic statistical concepts and statistical tests used in quantitative studies;
- plan quantitative data analysis;
- have some ideas about how to present and interpret your results;
- know what p values, confidence intervals, relative risk and odds ratios are.

Introduction

In this chapter we will explore approaches to quantitative data, offering some practical considerations on how to plan its analysis. We will introduce some basic concepts in statistics and statistical tests used in quantitative studies. This is at an introductory level and assumes no prior knowledge of this subject. We will not be looking at complex formulae, or deep maths and statistics, but we will be introducing you to the concepts you will see discussed in papers and which you will need to plan your own proposals. We will also look at some epidemiological measures of assessing risks of disease, and a means of assessing the clinical impact of experimental studies.

Analysing quantitative data

The focus of this section is to provide some understanding of the analytic procedures based upon descriptive and inferential statistics, which will enable you to discuss how you would go about analysing quantitative data in a research proposal.

Different levels of measurement of quantitative data

In order to be able to analyse quantitative data, it is necessary to understand that there are different levels of measurement inherent in different types of variables. Although this may initially appear slightly technical, it is necessary to understand these different types of data because they are treated differently. The different levels of measurement are as follows:

- Nominal (or categorical)-level data: data placed into named categories, such as male/female, which do not have a particular order. Although numbers may be used to code nominal data, these do not have arithmetical qualities. These are the most basic forms of data and not amenable to some forms of statistical analysis.
- Ordinal-level data: data placed into categories that have an order, a relationship with each other; for example, a Likert scale on a questionnaire in which the participant chooses from 'strongly agree', 'agree', 'neutral', 'disagree', 'strongly disagree'. We can infer the rank order but not the relative size. For example, we can infer that a participant who ticks 'strongly agree' holds the opinion more intensely than one who ticks 'agree'. However, we cannot infer whether, for example, the first participant feels twice or three times as strongly as the second, only the rank order or preference.
- Interval-level data: these are similar to ordinal data but ranked on a scale with equal intervals between categories (e.g. temperature). The scale does not have a zero-point anchored in the real world; for example, the Celsius scale has a zero point that is arbitrarily set at the temperature that water freezes. Interval data enable a wider range of mathematical procedures to be used.
- Ratio-level data: like interval-level data, but the categories have a scale with a true zero point, such as age or income. This is the highest level of data and enables a full range of mathematic procedures to be used.

Activity 7.1   Critical thinking

Imagine you are doing a research study into the drinking habits and satisfaction of different people in different pubs. Identify from the following those variables which are nominal, ordinal, interval and ratio:

- drinking alcohol: yes or no?
- number of alcoholic drinks consumed;
- satisfaction with the pub bar service ('very dissatisfied', 'dissatisfied', 'neutral', 'satisfied', 'very satisfied');

(Continued)

(Continued)

- number of men in the pub;
- number of women in the pub;
- income of each individual;
- pounds spent that evening;
- temperature in the bar area;
- would return: yes or no?
- eating food: yes or no?
- satisfaction with the pub food service ('very dissatisfied', 'dissatisfied', 'neutral', 'satisfied', 'very satisfied').

Answers are given at the end of the chapter.

Types of quantitative data analysis

Data can be analysed with descriptive and/or inferential statistics. Descriptive statistics are simply that: they describe the data. In many studies it is acceptable and correct only to use simple statistics like percentages or averages (means) to show the results, and conclusions can still be drawn from them. However, the growth in processing power of computers means that they are capable of running more complex operations. It has become possible for researchers to run more easily inferential statistics, and these functions are able to draw often sophisticated comparisons between variables in data. We will begin by looking at the different types of descriptive statistics that are available to you when analysing and presenting your data, and then move on to a brief indication of the types of inferential statistics that may be considered.

Simple descriptive statistics

Frequency tables enable you to show the incidence of particular responses. Percentages enable you to show figures as a proportion of the whole and can make data easier to understand.

What is the average? Measures of central tendency

Measures of central tendency report a typical or average value. The three main measures of central tendency are the mean, the median and the mode.

The *mean* is the arithmetic average, calculated by adding up the value of all of the responses and dividing by the number of responses received. It can only be used with interval and ratio data, which have true arithmetical properties. The *median* is the middle point when data are lined up in order. If you have an even number of data, it is halfway between the two middle values. The median can be used with any type of numerical data. The *mode* is the most common response given and can be used with all four types of data.

Since different questions produce different types of data (nominal, ordinal, ratio, and interval), you need to ensure that the measure of central tendency (mean, mode and median) is appropriate for the type of data you are collecting. If we apply this to Activity 7.1 above, we can see that the questionnaire produces nominal, ordinal and ratio data, which should be treated differently.

Different types of data

Nominal data

The question on drinking alcohol produces nominal data because, although numerical codes are given (yes = 1, no = 2), the data do not have arithmetical qualities. The mean cannot be used because it would be meaningless to calculate an 'average of whether drinking alcohol or not' of 1.5.

Ordinal data

The questions using Likert scales to measure whether drinkers are satisfied or not with the bar and food service produce ordinal data. If more pub goers were satisfied with the bar service than any of the other responses, the mode could be used to analyse these data, and if the scales were coded 1 for very dissatisfied up to 5 for very satisfied, the mode would be 4. It would, however, be inappropriate to work out a mean score because these are ordinal data and therefore do not have full numerical qualities; that is, the score 2 (= dissatisfied) is not twice the size of the score 4 (= satisfied).

Ratio data

The questions about the pub goers' incomes, numbers of drinks and pounds spent produce ratio data that have full numerical qualities (e.g. someone spending £20 spends twice as much as someone spending £10). Consequently, it would be appropriate to work out the mean by dividing the total sum of the spending with the number of respondents. So, for example, if total spending was £1,000 that evening and there were 100 people in the pub, the mean would be £10. The mode and median are also appropriate measures. In this example, let's assume there is no mode because no response appears more than once, but a median could be calculated. This would be done by lining up all the responses in numerical order and seeing which is the middle figure. Here is how it would be if there were 11 responses. The figures are the spending of each person in pounds:

5, 6, 8, 10, 15, 16, 17, 19, 24, 27, 29

The median is 16 because once the responses are lined up in numerical order, 16 is the middle response. Note the mean here is also 16. Medians may be used where extremes of data are in

(Continued)

(Continued)

evidence as the mean is more sensitive to extremes. For example, imagine we had received these responses:

1, 6, 8, 10, 15, 16, 17, 19, 24, 47, 59

Now, the median is still 16, but the mean has shifted to 20.18 in response to the more extreme values.

Table 7.1 summarises appropriate descriptive statistics for different levels of measurement.

Table 7.1 Appropriate descriptive statistics for different levels of measurement

	Mode	Median	Mean
Nominal	✓	✗	✗
Ordinal	✓	✓	✗
Interval	✓	✓	✓
Ratio	✓	✓	✓

What is the range? Measures of dispersion

Measures of dispersion indicate the degree of variety or spread of the data. Providing averages can be helpful for understanding the midpoint of data, but it is also important to look at the spread. The simplest way is using the range, which gives the lowest and highest points. Using the first set of data for pub spending from the box above, the mean is 16, but the range is 5–29. However, this simple range only gives the first and last points, and is unreliable concerning the variability of the data, so the interquartile range can be used (Parahoo, 2014) so that, using the median value again as a middle point (Q2, below), the data set can be analysed as quartiles (split into quarters). Using the data set from above for pounds spent, it can be analysed as quartiles like this:

5, 6, 8, 10, 15, 16, 17, 19, 24, 27, 29

↓ ↓   ↓

Q1 Q2 Q3

The interquartile range is the distance between the first and third quartiles, 8–24 (24 − 8 = 16). The semi-interquartile range is half the difference between Q1 and Q3, and in this example would be 16/2 = 8. This is the typical distance of scores from the median and is a more useful measure in describing the data set as it goes beyond either the median or the range (Parahoo, 2014).

The most frequently used measure for describing a data set is the *standard deviation* (SD), which shows an average of how all data points differ from the mean. In our pub spending example, if the spending of each individual was relatively similar (homogene-ous), then the SD would be small, zero or close to zero. If there was a great discrepancy between the pounds spent by all the pub goers (if their spending was relatively dissimi-lar or heterogeneous), then the SD would be larger. The exact SD will depend on all the values collected which form the data set and will be reported with the mean value.

Normal distribution

Normal distribution is a concept that has been demonstrated to be correct and forms part of central limit theorem. It applies to many human properties, such as intelligence quotient (IQ) measurement, height and weight, and students' test scores, where most people's scores are close to the mean value, with fewer scoring extreme values. A nor-mal distribution curve is a 'bell-shaped' curve (Figure 7.1), and it is important because many statistical tests rely on the assumption that data collected adhere to this relation-ship. In a normal distribution, 68 per cent of data will fall between 1 SD of the mean, 95 per cent of data will fall within 2 SD of the mean, 99.7 per cent of data will fall within 3 SD of the mean and 28 per cent will fall between 1 and 2 SD.

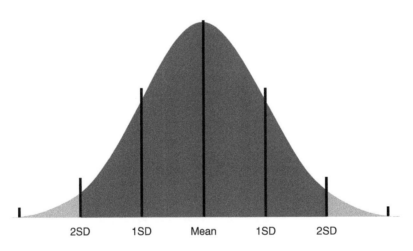

Figure 7.1 Normal distribution curve. Adapted from an original graph by Jeremy Kemp (2 September 2005)

Representing the results

The final part of data analysis is representing the results in an acceptable manner. In the descriptive statistics discussed above, frequency tables, simple graphs and pie charts could be used.

Frequency tables (like Table 7.2) present information about the relative occurrence of different values. They are useful when information is difficult to present in graph form because the highest and lowest values are significantly different, or a high level of preci-sion is required.

Overall, how satisfied are you with the bar service at this pub?

Table 7.2 Frequency table

	n	Per cent
Very dissatisfied	6	12%
Dissatisfied	24	48%
Neutral	11	22%
Satisfied	6	12%
Very satisfied	3	6%
Total	50	100%

Please note that the n column in Table 7.2 indicates the actual number of responses. This enables the reader to know how many responses were received and whether there were missing data. You can see from this table that this pub is not doing very well with its bar service, as 60 per cent are either dissatisfied or very dissatisfied.

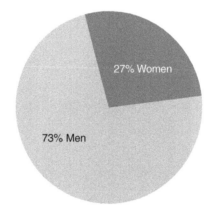

Figure 7.2 Pie chart

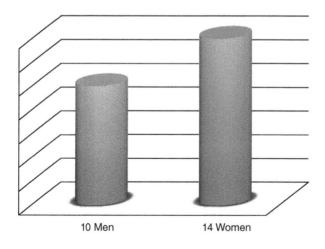

Figure 7.3 Bar graph

Pie charts enable you to present information about the relative proportion of different elements. They can be used when the values are added together, or you have only one set of data that all have positive values. You can see from the pie chart shown in Figure 7.2 that there were 73 per cent men in the pub, compared to 27 per cent women.

Bar graphs (Figure 7.3) enable you to compare data across categories. Simple bar graphs present single values and clustered bar graphs present groups of values together. In the example shown in Figure 7.3, comparing men's and women's dissatisfaction with bar service, you can see that women were more dissatisfied than men.

Inferential statistics

Descriptive statistics can be acceptable, but more interesting and important relationships can be uncovered between variables in quantitative studies using inferential statistics. It is here that hypotheses become particularly relevant, as they are tested using inferential statistics. If we have a null hypothesis, this means that there is no difference between variables, and the results are said to accept or reject that null hypothesis.

It is important to understand that inferential statistics are about estimating parameters or results in sample data. In research studies we are rarely able to gain data from an entire population, so we must sample them. Thus, we may select 1,000 people to represent a population of 1,000,000, as this would be cheaper, easier and more feasible given research-funding limitations. The purpose of inferential statistical testing is therefore to give us an idea of the relationships between variables that exist in our sample, and whether these might be expected to hold true in the wider population from which the sample was drawn.

Statistical significance

Statistical significance is said to be present by convention if a test gives a value of $p < 0.05$. What this means is that there is a less than 5 per cent chance of the results shown in the study sample being by chance, if they were repeated in the population; 5 per cent is taken as an acceptable level of probability although others can be set. $p < 0.01$ would be a 1 per cent chance (better); $p < 0.001$ would be a 0.01 per cent chance (even better) of the results in the study being by accident. The p value can be between 0 and 1 and is an index of the probability of the study results being likely if the study was repeated in a population. It works inversely, meaning that smaller is better. The p value does not tell us whether the study is a good one or not. Finding that there are no relationships between variables can be as interesting and relevant as finding that there are relationships. It is possible, however, that errors can be made in hypothesis testing. These can be type I and type II errors. A type I error occurs when a statistically significant relationship is found in a study where in fact it does not exist, and this might happen if the p value was set too high, hence the convention of $p < 0.05$. A type II error exists when no relationship is found when there is one. Either type of error can lead to the wrong conclusions being drawn about a study's results (Parahoo, 2014). (Please review the section on 'Sample size and power calculations' in Chapter 6 of this book, page 115, where the importance of sample size and power have already been discussed.)

Another way of estimating statistical significance is using CIs. These are ranges generated in the data from our sample between which we can be confident that the true value for the actual population will lie. By convention this is usually set at 95 per cent (although you may see 99 per cent CIs), meaning that our data will generate a range of values between which we can be 95 per cent certain that the true population value lies.

In Figure 7.4, the CIs are the lines which represent a range of values. The point estimates (or summary statistics) are the dots in the middle of the lines which indicate where the values for the actual population are estimated to lie. CIs will be in the units of the study (so if we were using them in our pub analogy, the units might be pints of beer). If the summary statistic (or point estimate) falls between the CIs, then we can be 95 per cent certain that these results represent the population and are statistically significant; if the summary statistic is outside the CIs, it is not statistically significant (Forster et al., 2014; Peat, 2002). CIs also allow us to assess the relative precision available in the results as the wider the CI, the less precise or less accurate an estimation the results are said to be. This can be related to sample size, so studies with larger samples may have narrower CIs than smaller studies, indicating that the larger samples give greater precision in the results. This can indicate which of the studies' results may be more clinically significant as larger studies with more precise results.

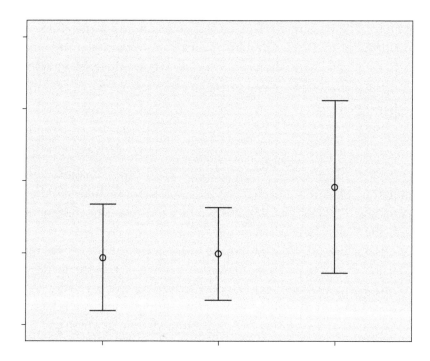

Figure 7.4   Confidence intervals containing point estimates. The right-hand one is a less precise estimate as it has a larger range. Adapted from an original graph by Sigbert (8 December 2008)

Deciding which statistical tests to use

In a real research project it would be necessary to obtain the help of a statistician on elements of statistical testing such as which tests to use. Local NHS Trusts usually have a research design service as part of their Research and Development Departments and statisticians should be available for consultation through them. For a proposal, you would be expected to identify your variables and the types of tests you would want to use. Obviously as you have not collected any data at this proposal stage you cannot actually run any tests. Some basic considerations in choosing which tests to use are listed in the box below.

If the data are normally distributed and the data are at interval/ratio level, then parametric statistics (which are more robust and powerful) can be used; if not, non-parametric tests are necessary (Peat, 2002). *Parametric* means that the data conform to certain assumptions, one of which is that they are normally distributed. This can be plotted in a distribution curve like the one in Figure 7.1 so that most of the data clusters around the mean, with more extreme values on the outer fringes. If data were plotted that looked exactly like Figure 7.1, they would be said to be normally distributed, but if there was a tendency for the data to cluster to the right or left of the mean, it would be said to be skewed.

Box 7.1: Deciding on which tests to use (adapted from Peat (2002))

1. If there is only one outcome variable
With interval/ratio variables, the following tests could be used:
   - one-sample *t*-tests, paired *t*-tests (if the variable was measured at more than one point in time), analysis of variance (if measured three or more times)

   With nominal-level variables:
   - proportions and CIs
   - McNemar's test (non-parametric, if the variables are measured more than once)
2. If there are two variables
With both interval/ratio variables:
   - Pearson's *r* correlation (parametric), regression

   With both nominal-level variables:
   - chi-squared, odds ratios

   With one nominal and one interval-level variable:
   - Spearman's rho (ρ) (non-parametric correlation), logistic regression, two-sample *t*-tests, Wilcoxon test, 95 per cent CIs
3. If there are more than two variables
   - multiple regression, analysis of variance (ANOVA), factor analysis

Applications

How might these types of statistics be used in study design?

Case study 7.1: Using statistical analysis

Imagine that we are researchers working for a cosmetics company. We have developed a new type of face cream that has cost millions of pounds to get to the stage of testing on humans. As part of that process, we decide to test the theory (hypothesis) that as we age we get more wrinkly.

In order to test the hypothesis, that as we age we get more wrinkly, we develop a measure of wrinkles, and use it on the faces of 1,000 volunteers. Next, we run a statistical test looking at the correlations between age and wrinkliness. A correlation is a measure of association. It does not prove that one variable causes another, but indicates instead that they are associated in some way.

The independent variable is age, the dependent is wrinkliness (we know this to be true as there is no way it could be the other way around: wrinkliness cannot cause ageing).

As the data are found to be normally distributed and at ratio level, we use Pearson's r correlation. We enter the data into the computer program SPSS, and test age against wrinkliness. The test will give us an absolute value for r as well as a p value. The value of r shows us the strength of association. (It varies between 0 and 1, with closest to 1 being strongest. It can be negative, indicating an inverse association, which would mean that in this example, as we age we get less wrinkly!) Statistical significance is said to be present by convention if a test gives a value of $p < 0.05$. What this means is that there is a less than 5 per cent chance of the results shown in the study sample being by chance. If the tests were run again with samples from the same population, 95/100 of the results would be the same. As we worked out in advance that the sample size was sufficient and our study was adequately powered (it had enough people in it to avoid errors), we can now say that as we age we get more wrinkly and that there is a strong correlation (as $r = +0.990$). We could also plot this on a scatter graph (Figure 7.5), and this plot would describe a line close to a left-to-right ascending diagonal line.

Next, we might decide to test our cream on different people. We assess the necessary sample size, recruit a random sample of people and then randomise them into a treatment and a control group. The treatment group will get our new cream, the control will get simple aqueous cream and the study will be double-blinded (neither researchers nor participants know whether they are getting the treatment or control cream). A baseline wrinkle measurement is taken at the start, participants are asked to use the creams for a month and then our investigators will reassess their wrinkles. We test the composition of each group at baseline to make sure that there were no biases in them; for example, if we had all the wrinkliest people in one group this would be a source of bias. At the end of the month, we want to see if there are statistically significant differences between the groups, and this would be our hypothesis (the null hypothesis being that there are no differences between the groups; technically, then, we are trying to reject the null hypothesis to demonstrate that there are differences between groups).

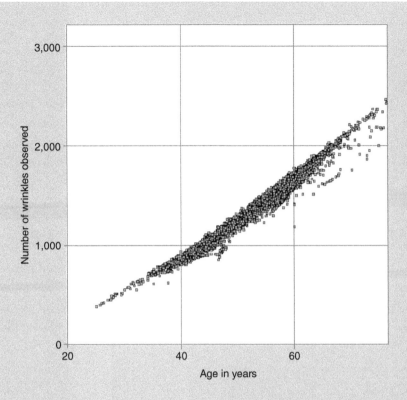

Figure 7.5 Scatterplot: this shows a strong positive correlation between age and wrinkles. Adapted from an original graph by Lars Aronsson (8 December 2008)

We would use an unpaired or 'independent samples' *t*-test as the data are at ratio level, demonstrated (by us) to be normally distributed, and this test will compare means from each group (if we were able to compare data from each actual participant, we could use a paired *t*-test). Using *t*-tests will give a value for the *t*-test and a *p* value, but the variables will be different from those mentioned above for correlations. In experimental designs, the independent variable will be the group into which participants are placed (treatment or control group creams) and the dependent variable will be the effect that each has on the wrinkles. So, in order to demonstrate that our new cream was effective, we would want to see a statistically significant difference ($p < 0.05$) between the two groups. If that was the case, we could report that the new cream was effective in reducing the number of wrinkles. We could also calculate CIs to give us the range of values of the means of the reduction in wrinkles in each group, and the size of this would indicate the relative accuracy of the results. For example, if the 95 per cent CI for the treatment groups was 850–950 (this means that our measure of wrinkliness shows that the range is between 850 and 950 wrinkles per face) and the summary statistic was 900, this is a more accurate estimate than if the 95 per cent CI for the control group was 500–2,500 wrinkles per face and the point estimate (or summary statistic) was 1,000.

We might think about being a bit more sophisticated with our analysis, and look at the impact that variables like age, sex, race, exposure to sunlight, location in the UK, smoking and so on

(Continued)

(Continued)

might have on the outcomes of our study. In that case, as well as stratifying our sampling to reflect these properties at the outset, we could use an ANOVA technique, which would compare the means of these different variables and give us an indication of the relative importance of each. There are many different varieties of ANOVA, and we'd definitely want a statistician involved if we were planning to use one of these. Their advantage is that if we were to try to analyse each variable in a series of single comparisons, there is a danger of getting type I errors, as we would need to test so many times that occasionally one would occur by chance.

Assessing risk and clinical significance

Studies may or may not demonstrate statistical significance, but this is a different concept to that of clinical significance. Risk can be assessed using epidemiological measures such as the relative risk (RR) and odds ratios (OR), which are used to describe the risk of contracting a disease. Number needed to treat (NNT) shows the clinical impact of treatment outcomes (Peat, 2002).

Relative risk

This describes associations between exposures and outcomes in prospective studies rather than case-control studies. It is quite a simple concept, where the rate of an illness in the exposed group is compared with that in the unexposed group. This could be used, for example, to show the RR to smokers of contracting lung cancer compared to non-smokers. It is time-dependent, as there are time factors associated with it, such as the time it takes to develop lung cancer (Peat, 2002). The results will be expressed by calculating CIs around a point estimate.

Odds ratios

These are not time-dependent and can be used in case-control studies where the proportions of cases and controls are limited because the sampling methods employed in the study mean that the prevalence of the disease in the study is not the same as the prevalence in the population. OR is similar to RR but not the same, and is calculated differently, giving the odds of contracting a disease. Thus, the OR for contracting lung cancer if one is a smoker is different from the RR because the RR gives the risk of a person who is a smoker contracting lung cancer, while the OR shows the likelihood that a person with lung cancer has been a smoker. CIs around a point estimate will be calculated here too. If the range given by the CI includes 1.0 then the effect is not statistically significant, as 1.0 indicates that there is no RR or OR in one group compared to another (Peat, 2002). This is particularly useful if we have more than one factor involved in our analysis, as it can be drawn in a graph known as a forest plot (or 'blobbogram') and different results compared (Figure 7.6). It can also be used to compare and combine the results of individual studies (there is more in Chapter 8 on systematic reviews and meta-analyses).

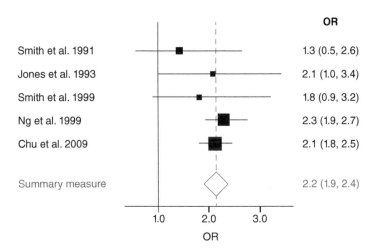

Figure 7.6   Forest plot: this shows confidence intervals, point estimates as black boxes and a summary measure in the larger diamond. OR odds ratio. Reproduced from an original graph by Jimjamjak (4 May 2010)

In the example in Figure 7.6, to the left of the figure is the name of each individual study, the lines next to them are the CIs and the black boxes are the point estimates. You can see that in these studies Smith et al. (1991 and 1999) all overlap 1.0 so the effect is probably not statistically significant, even though the point estimate is greater than 1.0. Jones et al. (1993), Ng et al. (1999) and Chu et al. (2009) are less ambiguous as they do not cross 1.0. The overall odds ratio (the diamond) here is 2.0, meaning that the odds of having the disease in question (whatever it may be) are twice as great if a patient is exposed to some predisposing factor. (If Figure 7.6 represented smoking we could say that a patient with lung cancer is twice as likely, based on these studies, to be a smoker, but as the studies in this figure are not about lung cancer don't quote that.)

Number needed to treat

This can be calculated from RCTs and indicates how many patients would need to receive the new treatment for one additional patient to benefit (Peat, 2002). It allows for comparisons between treatments of their clinical effectiveness and cost-effectiveness, as a treatment that saves one additional life for every ten patients treated is better than one that saves one additional life for every 100 patients treated. If they cost the same, then the first treatment is the most cost-effective. NNT is calculated by finding the absolute risk reduction (ARR) of each treatment and subtracting them (Peat, 2002). So, if one treatment reduces risk by 10 per cent and another by 15 per cent, 15 − 10 = 5 per cent or 0.05 ARR. NNT = 1/ARR, or 1/0.05 = 20. This shows that 20 patients will need to take the new treatment to prevent one death. CIs would also be calculated for NNT.

Chapter summary

In this chapter we have explored approaches to quantitative data and offered some practical considerations on how to plan their analysis. We have introduced some basic concepts in statistics and statistical tests used in quantitative studies, and some ideas about how data can be presented and interpreted. We have looked at descriptive and inferential statistics, p values and CIs, RR, OR and NNT.

Activity: Brief outline answer

Activity 7.1   Critical thinking (page 129–30)

- Drinking alcohol: yes or no? Nominal data
- Number of alcoholic drinks consumed: ratio data
- Satisfaction with the pub bar service: ordinal data
- Number of men in the pub: ratio data
- Number of women in the pub: ratio data
- Income of each individual: ratio data
- Pounds spent that evening: ratio data
- Temperature in the bar area: interval data
- Would return: yes or no? Nominal data
- Eating food: yes or no? Nominal data
- Satisfaction with the pub food service: ordinal data

Further reading

Cullum, N, Ciliska, D, Haynes, RB and Marks, S (2008) *Evidence-Based Nursing: An Introduction.* Oxford: Blackwell Publishing.

Lots of relevant chapters on understanding and interpreting concepts discussed in this chapter.

De Vaus, DA (2014) *Surveys in Social Research* (6th edition). London: Routledge.

Classic text on surveys that provides a good overview of the process.

Forster, L, Diamond, I and Banton, J (2014) *Beginning Statistics: An Introduction for Social Scientists* (2nd edition). London: Sage.

Background reading

Maltby, J, Day, L and Williams, G (2007) *Introduction to Statistics for Nurses.* Harlow: Pearson Education.

Very good background reading on statistics.

Parahoo, K (2014) *Nursing Research: Principles, Process and Issues* (3rd edition). Basingstoke: Palgrave Macmillan.

Good, readable background information on study design and quantitative data analysis.

Peat, J (2002) *Health Science Research: A Handbook of Quantitative Methods, Part 6: Analysing the Data.* London: Sage.

Very good on the subject of which statistical tests to use and more depth than presented here.

Sapsford, R (2007) *Survey Research* (2nd edition). London: Sage.

A readable and useful guide to survey research.

Useful websites

http://statpages.org

Web pages that perform statistical calculations from Statpages.org. Links and calculating pages.

www.ats.ucla.edu/stat/mult_pkg/whatstat/default.htm

University of California, Los Angeles guide to which statistics to use and how to run them in various computer packages.

Chapter 8 — Using and critiquing systematic reviews and meta-analyses

Chapter aims

After reading this chapter, you should be able to:

- explain the rationale for systematic reviews and meta-analyses;
- construct a protocol for a systematic review and meta-analysis;
- understand which quantitative and qualitative techniques are used in meta-analysis;
- have some understanding of how to critically appraise systematic reviews and meta-analyses;
- explain the role of the Cochrane Collaboration and similar bodies;
- describe how systematic reviews and meta-analyses inform the production of clinical guidelines and the work of NICE and SIGN.

Introduction

Having examined in previous chapters quantitative and qualitative research designs and their data analysis relating to single empirical studies, we will now move on to looking at how these can be amalgamated in systematic reviews (SRs) and meta-analyses. We are looking now at a secondary research technique, having spent much of the preceding pages looking at primary research studies and their designs. This is a comparatively recent development in nursing research, which has its roots in analysing experimental designs for medical decision making and has now become an important global movement. It is essentially a simple idea: if lots of studies have been done in a broadly similar area, why not combine them and produce an overall result? Hence it is a secondary technique, as a primary research study is a single study in which empirical data have been collected in that study, whereas in a systematic review and meta-analysis the authors are using the data reported in other people's studies. SRs are a scientific research activity in themselves (Clarke, 2006), in which reviewers search out and include all papers relevant to a predefined question, and then combine them using statistical methods to produce a summary finding, like a 'headline', which is frequently a recommendation for healthcare decision making and/or changes in practice. Statistical techniques (for quantitative studies) or discussion (for qualitative work) give an overview (meta-analysis) of the key issues. Predefined questions are addressed using methodologies made explicit before the review starts, so that the studies discovered are included or excluded by relevant criteria so that elements of bias are ruled out (Clarke, 2006). One major flaw with *non-systematic* reviews is the extent to which researchers can include studies which give a biased picture of evidence that can be made to support their own views and so this systematic approach removes this (Hemingway and Brereton, 2009). You will rarely see non-systematic reviews of literature published in good-quality journals nowadays.

Rapid reviews, in which authors are commissioned to undertake a rapid assessment of the literature, making sure that 'users' (patients, clients, carers) are involved, are recent trends (Hemingway and Brereton, 2009) which seek to make SRs relevant and responsive to changing healthcare demands. They may be less exhaustive than full systematic reviews and might be called scoping reviews.

The chapter begins by outlining the rationale for SRs and meta-analyses, and how to construct a protocol for an SR and meta-analysis. We will then go on to introduce some relevant quantitative and qualitative techniques. We will look at how SRs might be critiqued using a CASP tool. We will look at the work of the Cochrane Collaboration and other bodies, and then at how SRs and meta-analyses inform the production of clinical guidelines and the work of NICE and other similar bodies.

Rationale for systematic reviews and meta-analyses

Mulrow (1995) outlines several key reasons why SRs are valuable as a scientific activity which aids healthcare decision making.

Box 8.1: Rationale for systematic reviews, adapted from Mulrow (1995)

1. Large quantities of information are available in many healthcare fields and this needs to be condensed and refined into manageable units that can be explored critically and key findings need to be disseminated in an intelligible format.

(Continued)

(Continued)

2. As well as clinicians using SRs for decision making, researchers and policy makers use them for purposes such as economic evaluation, refining of hypotheses, sample sizes and variables.

3. Although time-consuming and exacting to carry out, SRs are usually cheaper and easier to undertake than large-scale studies that address and overcome flaws and limitations in previous studies. Updating SRs can lead to a better understanding of issues as well as refining effect sizes. Mulrow (1995) quotes the example of streptokinase (a thrombolytic or clot-busting drug used to save lives post myocardial infarction) which, if relevant SRs had been updated as new studies became available, would have been shown to be effective 20 years earlier than when definitive evidence was available from primary studies.

4. Generalisability can be effectively assessed from SRs, as contextual information can be taken into account which can overcome the local context of studies that may have different eligibility criteria, disease definitions and study designs.

5. Consistency of relationships can be established. SRs can show that findings from several studies point in the same direction. In experimental designs, the magnitude and direction of treatments can be indicated, or in qualitative studies a narrative can be constructed which indicates the overall themes from each study. Similarly, SRs can also indicate inconsistencies and conflicts in the data.

6. Quantitative SRs can establish power and precision, meaning that the statistical analyses from several studies can be combined to give a more authoritative statistical meta-analysis when the studies are pooled, and estimates of effect sizes can become more precise. We will examine how this is done in more detail later.

7. Accuracy: by using explicit scientific principles for the inclusion and exclusion of studies, SRs overcome the potential bias associated with non-systematic reviews, which is the danger that researchers include evidence that only supports their own theoretical position.

In addition, Hemingway and Brereton (2009) add that SRs can give authoritative 'headline' findings for use in healthcare decision making; are increasingly a requirement of undergraduate and postgraduate research work; and are central to the NICE health technology assessment process for technology appraisals and the production of clinical guidelines.

Writing a proposal for a systematic review

A proposal for an SR is usually known as a protocol. While most institutions will want you to write a proposal for an empirical primary research study, some may allow you to construct an SR instead.

Khan et al. (2011) outline a five-stage approach:

1. framing questions for a review;
2. identifying the relevant literature;
3. assessing the quality of the literature;
4. summarising the evidence;
5. interpreting the findings.

Stage 1: Framing questions for a review

Rather than PICO, which we looked at in Chapter 2, Khan et al. (2011) use the mnemonic PIOS – **p**opulation, **i**ntervention (or **e**xposure), **o**utcomes and **s**tudy designs (suitable for addressing the questions). This will allow you to design a structured question as well as indicate which types of study design are suitable for answering your question. Questions asking for information on 'what works best?' are likely to be answered by experimental designs, whereas questions asking, 'what are patients' experience of illness?' are likely to be best answered by qualitative designs.

Stage 2: Identifying relevant literature

We have already discussed issues in literature searching. In an SR protocol, you must show that you plan to be thorough and exhaustive, and present a review plan that is free from bias and transparent in being able to find everything that has been published in an area. You will want to outline a large number of search terms, exploring the topic from many different angles, as well as listing all the databases you will search and including Cochrane and NICE guidelines. You should have a plan for dealing with grey literature (unpublished material, conference presentations that are not published as articles, PhD theses) and be ready to e-mail authors and scour reference lists for material not identified in other ways. You need to reconcile sensitivity with precision: a review that is 100 per cent sensitive to every possible paper is likely to be quite imprecise and so you are likely to get lots of papers not directly relevant to the subject. A precise search may run the risk of missing papers which do not exactly fit the search terms but will give you a smaller number of papers to review. Publication bias is also an issue: smaller studies or studies with non-significant results are less likely to be published, so it is possible that studies you find, when meta-analysed, overestimate the extent to which the new treatment or intervention is effective. Once you have searched your databases using multiple search terms, you will need to apply inclusion and exclusion criteria, and these should be stated in advance. This extraction of papers is crucial to getting appropriate evidence and is known as screening.

Stage 3: Assessing the quality of the literature

Critiquing research reports and giving a critical appraisal of a body of literature are large topics in themselves. In a protocol you should outline what criteria are to be used.

It is unlikely that you'll develop these yourself, and appropriate frameworks such as those given for primary studies on the NHS CASP website (**https://casp-uk.net**) will be useful for you. Specialist organisations such as the Cochrane Collaboration have their own frameworks that reviewers use for quality assessment and, whilst these are authoritative, they require training so it is unlikely that you will use them for undergraduate work. More than one person should independently screen and review the retrieved searches as an additional step in rigour in SRs. The quality of studies is frequently assessed and given numerical values based on the criteria employed. Reviewers should agree a cut-off point for inclusion of studies and discuss and agree independently which ones should be included and why. A summary of the papers included and excluded, and the criteria used should be given: a useful tool for showing this is the flow diagram from PRISMA (**www.prisma-statement.org**), which can be downloaded as a Word document.

Stage 4: Summarising the evidence

We discuss issues in meta-analyses in qualitative, quantitative and mixed-method SRs in more detail below. In your protocol you should outline exactly how this will be done, including some reference to the relative heterogeneity and how it might be tested (in quantitative reviews) or otherwise accounted for (in qualitative ones). In all reviews, but particularly in mixed-method ones, you may also have methodological heterogeneity (Khan et al., 2011). This may make combining studies difficult, but their findings can still be contrasted and assessed.

Stage 5: Interpreting the findings

If you are writing a protocol, you won't have any interpretation to do, but the key issues are as follows (Khan et al., 2011):

- Are the searches adequate? Is it clear that the search has been thorough, transparent, and free from bias?
- Are there publication biases? This occurs when the outcome of a study influences whether it will be published. For example, studies that show that an intervention is ineffective may be less likely to be published. Funnel plots can be used to indicate publication bias.
- Is the quality of the included studies high enough? This will be derived from your critical appraisal of the included studies. It may be that the quality of the studies is such that they cannot be meta-analysed.
- Are any outcomes clinically significant? Are changes in policy and practice necessary, and are new approaches to research required?

While the processes of systematically searching, including/excluding papers and reviewing the literature are broadly similar, quantitative, and qualitative techniques, meta-analysis and synthesis of the literature are quite different. We will now go on to examine these key differences.

You will find many examples of software that you can use to make authorative systematic review. One of the most impressive is that from the Joanna Briggs Institute (JBI). JBI SUMARI facilitates the process from protocol to report and allows team management for collaboration. JBI also provides critical appraisal tools covering all aspects of research appraisal. They are similar in intent to those of CASP but are different in content. You would need training and a subscription for JBI software, so it would not be suitable for individual or small studies, but some universities provide access for postgraduates. Cochrane provides RevMan but again this is a complex tool. Rayyan is free to use for people just starting out and might be an option for small student projects.

Quantitative systematic reviews and meta-analyses

If the initial research question is about 'what works best?' and there are clear comparisons between an active treatment (or intervention) and a control (or usual care), then study designs in the papers retrieved will include experimental, quasi-experimental and cohort studies. The aims of meta-analysis in this case are to estimate an overall effect size and whether the effect is roughly similar or dissimilar in different settings. This can be summarised in a narrative form if the papers are relatively heterogeneous (dissimilar), meaning that the papers are discussed rather than statistically analysed (NHS Centre for Reviews and Dissemination (NHS CRD), 2006). If the studies are relatively homogeneous (similar), they can be combined statistically. If possible, the measurements used in the studies can be used to pool their results, and usually this is presented for an intervention as the extent to which change was affected. This is presented differently if the data are in binary or continuous form. Odds ratios can be used if the data are binary, but these can overestimate treatment effects. Differences in means or standardised mean differences (d-statistics, z-scores and effect sizes) are used if the data are continuous (NHS CRD, 2006).

Results are usually presented in a forest plot (so called because it can look a bit like a tree). If we turn back to Figure 7.6 (page 143), where we looked at how odds ratios are presented, the format of this figure is similar to the presentation of statistical meta-analysis. For the purposes of meta-analysis, however, the line 1.0 is used to assess the effectiveness of treatment, so studies to the left of 1.0 on the graph indicate that the active treatment is better, whereas those to the right of the line indicate that the active treatment is worse. This will be clearly indicated in the forest plots reported in SRs. In Figure 7.6 we can also see that the studies have received a weighting, and this is represented by how large the effect size box is drawn. We can see that Jones et al. (1993, 1999) have relatively small effect sizes whereas Ng et al. (1999) and Chu et al. (2009) have much bigger boxes. This weighting takes into account the relative size of the study, with the largest studies receiving the largest weighting as represented in the confidence intervals (CIs): the narrower the CI the larger the study in terms of patient number and the greater the precision in the result. So, we can see that, as 1.0 = no difference between the active or control groups, and the summary effect size diamond = 2.0, the active treatment is worse than the control in this example.

Concept summary 8.1

This is a bit advanced for undergraduate work but might be useful for postgraduates.

Fixed and random effects models

Fixed effects models ignore the studies' heterogeneity and assume that the treatment effects are consistent across studies. Random effects models assume that other factors may modify treatment effects, are usually more conservative in their estimation of confidence intervals and can give too much weight to smaller studies, whereas fixed effects models may produce too precise treatment effects. Methods used in each are Mantel–Haenszel and Peto odds ratios and means for fixed effects models; random effect models use DerSimonian and Laird, and Bayesian models. These are quite complex terms, and you are not expected to do much more at this level than recognise them as types of tests used in statistical meta-analysis. More information can be found in NHS CRD (2006).

Studies in a review can also be tested for heterogeneity, publication bias (using funnel plots) and sensitivity using sensitivity analysis: the latter indicates how robust the overall analysis is (NHS CRD, 2006). Testing for heterogeneity is important because, if the studies are too dissimilar, reviewers run the risk of combining things that are not alike. For example, if one trial used a new analgesic in only the postoperative period, should its findings be amalgamated with one in which the analgesic was continued for three months? If the first study used it in a dosage of 30 mg twice daily, can it be meta-analysed with one where 60 mg four times daily was used? What if the studies used different pain-scoring techniques? There are statistical tests used in testing for heterogeneity, including chi-squared and the I statistic. Authors should investigate heterogeneity and it should be reported, if not it is a serious limitation. If the studies retrieved are simply too dissimilar and statistical analysis is meaningless, then they can still be synthesised, but the authors would need to discuss their results in a written rather than statistical form, known as narrative synthesis.

Publication bias

Publication bias can be difficult to establish. In general, positive studies (studies that show something) are more likely to be published, even though non-statistically significant results may be just as clinically important as statistically significant ones. For example, it might be just as useful to know that a new and expensive drug does not work (and so should not be prescribed) as it is to know that it does work. Both are clinically important results. Such publication bias means that, if a literature search and subsequent meta-analysis were carried out, it would overstate the extent to which any new treatment or intervention had positive results. In theory, it should be possible to plot the results of each study in the review on a graph, and it should look like a pyramid (or funnel). If there is a bite or chunk missing from the funnel, this could indicate publication bias. In Figure 8.1, you can see a funnel plot with a good, nearly symmetrical spread of data. The points represent results in studies found by the reviewers. On the *x* (horizontal) axis would be the result statistics (for example, risk ratios) and on the *y* (vertical) axis would be sample size. In Figure 8.2 you can see the funnel plot redrawn with some of the small, inconclusive, or negative results omitted, as if the reviewers had not found them because they had not been published (or even suppressed). You can see in Figure 8.2 that there is a chunk missing, so the funnel plot is asymmetrical, indicating possible publication bias. Publication bias demonstrated like this might be something of a tentative finding because it may be that actually there are no studies to find (Gough et al., 2017).

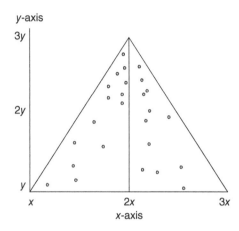

Figure 8.1   Generic funnel plot. Reproduced from an original graph by Nousernamesleft (21 January 2008). Made freely available for any purpose under the Wikimedia Creative Commons License via Wikipedia (see http://commons.wikimedia.org/wiki/Main_Page for further information)

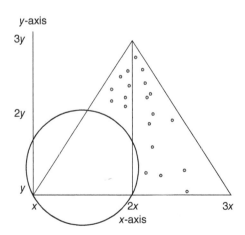

Figure 8.2   Funnel plot showing publication bias. Adapted from an original graph by Nousernamesleft (21 January 2008). Made freely available for any purpose under the Wikimedia Creative Commons License via Wikipedia (see http://commons.wikimedia.org/wiki/Main_Page for further information)

Authors of SRs may show funnel plots and should also convince you that they have gone to great lengths to find all possible studies, including unpublished studies, to overcome possible publication bias and make sure their meta-analysis conclusions are based on the widest available evidence.

Sensitivity analysis in a quantitative SR can be tested by removing the results of one or more studies from the analysis to examine the impact that this has on the meta-analysis. If there are a small number of studies, the overall synthesis might be dominated by one or two, so removing them can illustrate if this is the case and allow the reviewers to make judgements about the robustness of their analysis (Gough et al., 2017).

Qualitative systematic reviews and meta-analyses

As there has been a large growth in qualitative research in recent years, techniques have been developed which allow overviews of these studies to be constructed. While searching, including and reviewing studies will be similar processes, there can be no statistical meta-analysis as there would be with experimental designs. This leads qualitative researchers to use different terminology for their meta-analysis, and terms such as meta-study and meta-synthesis are used instead, as is the term meta-ethnography (Lloyd Jones, 2006). Some qualitative reviews will be largely descriptive, but generally they are interpretative in that they seek to synthesise a number of studies' findings and reinterpret them to give an overview of the body of literature and offer new insights and understandings which can provide a foundation for future research and advance thinking about key issues (Lloyd Jones, 2006).

One common criticism of qualitative research is that it does not produce generalisable findings, so it is much more difficult for the meaning of qualitative studies to be interpreted in different settings. However, if several qualitative studies could be combined, then the similarities and differences of the primary studies could be used to inform research and practice in that field. The rich, in-depth data gained from patients and service users is useful to understand patients' experiences of illness, service delivery and barriers to service usage (Ring et al., 2011) and so synthesis of qualitative studies is important.

Unlike quantitative meta-analysis, which can be accomplished in a relatively straightforward statistical manner if the studies are homogeneous, qualitative evidence synthesis is more tentative, exploratory and contested. This is an emerging field and there are a variety of different ways in which it can be done. Unless they take a generic qualitative approach, qualitative studies will have particular philosophical perspectives, and are very much derived from the context and subjective views of participants (Ring et al., 2011), meaning that one group of participants may give quite different views than another because their experiences might be entirely dissimilar. This does not mean that there is something wrong with qualitative research studies with conflicting findings, just that human beings can experience any aspect of the world very differently.

Although searching for studies ought to be as rigorous a process as in a quantitative SR, quality appraisal of qualitative studies is not straightforward and there is little consensus about what the criteria might be for high-quality qualitative studies (Ring et al., 2011).

It is beyond the scope of this book to detail the similarities and differences between qualitative evidence synthesis techniques; Ring et al. (2011) list the following methods:

- critical interpretive synthesis;
- grounded theory synthesis;
- meta-ethnography;
- meta-interpretation;
- meta-study;
- meta-summary;
- qualitative cross-case analysis;
- thematic synthesis.

In qualitative evidence synthesis, results are interpreted by reviewers. The studies may be quite different in their settings and contexts, but novel conceptualisations and extrapolations are drawn that go beyond the studies included (Lloyd Jones, 2006). Key features are outlined in the box below.

Box 8.2:   Key features of a meta-synthesis

Lloyd Jones (2006) gives the following as key features of a meta-synthesis:

1. Focus of study, inclusion and exclusion criteria and theoretical framework: rather than having a 'what works best?' question, the focus may be on broad areas or concepts, and may also be meaningful and relevant for healthcare decision making. Inclusion criteria may be about samples, settings and themes, and possibly methodologies.
2. Study identification: this will be by an exhaustive literature search, in the same way that any other review would be undertaken.
3. Study selection: this is a less precise field than in statistical meta-analysis, given that less precise criteria are used to assess the quality of qualitative studies. Once again, precision must be reconciled with sensitivity in the search.
4. Summary analysis and synthesis of findings: findings can be synthesised using formal techniques such as grounded formal theory and meta-ethnography, but less structured approaches of interpretation can also be used. Whichever methods are used should be clearly specified and transparent, with categories developed similar to themes and subthemes in primary studies, with an eye on uniqueness for emerging theories and

(Continued)

(Continued)

evidence which confirms and refutes them. Lots of different ways of analysing the data should be considered, and tabulation is important, meaning that the studies included should be grouped together in a table showing which themes are shared, confirmed, and refuted by using which studies. Date, geography, methodology and other categories can also be used to tabulate findings, but interpretations must be based on themes or theories that emerge rather than these already-existing categories.

5. Interpretation of results: this will depend on the field and initial question(s) and reviewers will need to tailor their work to their audiences.

Combining mixed methods studies in a systematic review

If a review is not driven by a clear 'what works?' question, it is likely that studies from multiple methodologies may be obtained. This will necessitate their review and meta-analysis using a combination of approaches, outlined above. This means that the interpretation will be more complex, but it is possible to compare findings of the different meta-analysis methods and use the insights gained from the different methodological approaches to triangulate the results of the review.

Cochrane Collaboration and other bodies

The Cochrane Collaboration

The Cochrane Collaboration (**www.cochrane.org**) is named after Archie Cochrane, an epidemiologist who pioneered the use of RCTs as a means of informing healthcare practice. It is an independent, not-for-profit organisation and receives funding from various sources, including governments, universities, hospital Trusts, charities and personal donations. It was established in 1993 as an international network and makes freely accessible Cochrane Reviews via its Library, which is searchable, free of charge.

Figure 8.3 is the logo of the Cochrane Collaboration. It incorporates a forest plot showing the meta-analysis of the use of corticosteroids with pregnant women to improve outcomes for their premature babies. The meta-analysis indicates that steroid usage improves outcomes, as the summary (the diamond) is to the left of the line. Outcomes were 30–50 per cent better when the mothers had been treated before birth with steroids. Changes in practice have resulted from this meta-analysis as it provides clear evidence of the clinical effectiveness of the treatment.

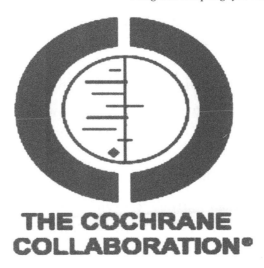

Figure 8.3 The Cochrane Collaboration logo. Used with permission from Nick Royle, CEO, the Cochrane Collaboration, Oxford, UK

The Joanna Briggs Institute

The Joanna Briggs Institute (**https://jbi.global**) is an international, not-for-profit research and development organisation within the Faculty of Health and Medical Sciences at the University of Adelaide. It makes accessible resources for evidence-based healthcare for nurses, midwives, medics and allied health professionals. It seeks to improve the health status of the global population through the delivery of evidence-based healthcare. This is achieved by developing methods to appraise and synthesise evidence and by conducting SRs and analyses of the research literature, as well as dissemination and implementation of evidence.

The Cochrane Nursing Care Field

The Cochrane Nursing Care Field (**https://nursing.cochrane.org**) was established in 2009 as a result of the initiative of nurses at the Joanna Briggs Institute in Australia. It has three functions related to the production and use of Cochrane reviews, which are: to support Cochrane in the preparation of reviews relevant to nursing; to introduce perspectives relevant to all those providing nursing care (nurses, other disciplines such as social work, families and lay caregivers); and to enhance the dissemination and effective uptake of Cochrane reviews.

NHS Institute for Health Research Centre for Reviews and Dissemination (CRD)

The CRD (**www.york.ac.uk/inst/crd**) is a department of the University of York and is part of the National Institute for Health Research. It is responsible for undertaking high-quality SRs to evaluate the effects of health and social care interventions and the delivery and organisation of healthcare.

Database of Abstracts of Reviews of Effects (DARE)

DARE (**www.crd.york.ac.uk/CRDWeb**) contains 15,000 abstracts of SRs, including over 6,000 quality-assessed reviews, as well as details of all Cochrane reviews and protocols.

NHS Economic Evaluation Database (EED)

NHS EED (**www.crd.york.ac.uk/CRDWeb**) contains 24,000 abstracts of health economics papers, including over 7,000 quality-assessed economic evaluations. It is aimed at decision makers and identifies, describes and appraises economic evaluations.

Health Technology Assessment (HTA) database

The HTA database (**www.crd.york.ac.uk/CRDWeb**) brings together and describes details of completed and ongoing health technology assessments from around the world.

Activity 8.1   Research and finding evidence, and critical thinking

This is likely to be a time-consuming activity and may need to be revisited and refined over a number of days, particularly in terms of your search questions, which is why there is only one activity in this chapter. Don't print the studies you find, just read the abstracts on screen. You can save the abstracts to a folder in your computer and return to them later on.

1. Using Khan et al.'s (2011) mnemonic PIOS (population, intervention, outcomes, study design), produce a question for yourself based on your clinical nursing interests.
2. Search all the databases given immediately above and write a list of the reviews you find. How many have you found? Are they similar? Are they the same reviews? Do they have similar findings and recommendations? How do these reviews compare to current practice in your area?
3. Next, frame the question differently so that it contains the phrase 'patients' experiences of'. Use your university library journal search database and Google Scholar. What kinds of papers are identified now? Ask yourself the same questions as in point 2, above. How do the results from these two sets of searches compare? Are there differences between the qualitative and quantitative literature?
4. Write a short synthesis of findings from each search. Is one methodology overwhelmingly represented in your results? Are there flaws you can identify in any of the studies? Are there consistencies or inconsistencies in the recommendations from each methodology? Are changes in practice required in your area?

This represents your assessment of this body of literature, so there is no answer at the end of the chapter.

How systematic reviews and meta-analyses inform the production of clinical guidelines

NICE and SIGN

NICE (**www.nice.org.uk**) provides guidance, sets quality standards and manages a national database to improve people's health and prevent and treat ill health. There is a searchable database on the website. NICE makes recommendations on:

- new and existing medicines, treatments and procedures;
- treating and caring for people with specific diseases and conditions;
- how to improve people's health and prevent illness and disease.

These recommendations from NICE guidelines are not compulsory, but they are a key aspect of standard setting and clinical governance throughout the NHS. NICE also works towards implementation and has specific implementation activities and plans to make sure research findings change practice.

The Scottish Intercollegiate Guidelines Network (SIGN: **www.sign.ac.uk**) undertakes similar activities for the NHS in Scotland. It commissions reviews of the literature and produces guidelines for Scotland with the aim of improving Scottish health, reducing variations in care, and disseminating best practice. There are broad similarities between NICE and SIGN.

NICE and SIGN use similar processes to an SR and meta-analysis to form conclusions and recommendations on particular clinical questions. An exhaustive search is carried out, studies are tabulated, and their quality assessed. Various methods of assessment can be used. It is common that papers will be judged using some form of hierarchy of evidence, as this means that different types of research and evidence can be given a weighting to indicate their importance, and the overall quality of the evidence assessed. In this, the clinical effectiveness of different study designs is assessed and those higher in the hierarchy gain greater weight. You'll see many different formulations of hierarchies of evidence, but all are reasonably similar. The one shown in Table 8.1 has been adapted from the University of Oxford Centre for Evidence-Based Medicine (CEBM: **www.cebm.net**) and relates to therapeutic interventions.

Table 8.1 Centre for Evidence-Based Medicine hierarchy of evidence (adapted from Howick (2009))

Level	Study design
1a	Systematic reviews and meta-analyses of randomised controlled trials (with homogeneity).
1b	Individual randomised controlled trials with narrow confidence intervals.

(Continued)

Table 8.1   (Continued)

Level	Study design
2a	Systematic reviews and meta-analyses of cohort studies* (with homogeneity).
2b	Individual cohort study.
3a	Systematic reviews and meta-analyses of case-control studies† (with homogeneity).
3b	Individual case-control studies.
4	Case series‡ or poor cohort or case-control studies.
5	Expert opinion.

*A cohort study is one in which one group of patients received an intervention and another did not, and they are followed to assess the outcomes. This is a pragmatic design, and patients are not recruited or randomised by the researchers.

†A case-control study is one in which patients are identified by outcome and compared to others without that outcome to assess whether they had the same exposure.

‡A case series study is one where patients are assessed for outcomes without a control or comparison group.

If this hierarchy was used for grading a body of literature and to make recommendations, as is frequently the case in NICE and SIGN guidelines, it would produce a grading strategy which looks like the one in Table 8.2. A set of guidelines with mostly grade A studies would have a robust evidence base and be suitable for recommending changes to clinical practice.

Table 8.2   Grading structure for recommendations (adapted from Howick, 2009)

Grade	Assessment
A	Mostly level 1 studies.
B	Consistently level 2 or 3 studies.
C	Level 4 studies.
D	Level 5 studies or inconsistent or inconclusive studies at any level.

This CEBM definition does not include any qualitative research in its assessment of the effectiveness of different study designs. Some authors publish hierarchies of evidence which include qualitative studies; for example, Moule and Goodman (2016) present and discuss a model adapted from various sources which shows qualitative work as rating at level 4 in a hierarchy of evidence. Daly et al. (2007) propose a separate hierarchy for qualitative work (Table 8.3), although this is yet to be widely accepted by bodies such as NICE and SIGN.

Daly et al.'s (2007) ideas are controversial in that many qualitative researchers would strongly dispute the relevance of the concept of generalisability in relation to their work. Quantitative researchers and those conducting RCTs might also argue that it is impossible to tell the impact or effectiveness of most qualitative studies as they contain no measurements, but this is to reopen well-rehearsed arguments which we were at pains to move beyond in Chapter 1.

Table 8.3 Hierarchy of evidence for qualitative work (adapted from Daly et al., 2007)

Level	Study design
I	Generalisable studies*
II	Conceptual studies†
III	Descriptive studies‡
IV	Single-case studies§

*Generalisable studies are those with an extensive literature review which build on strong theoretical and methodological frameworks.

†Conceptual studies are those where a clear conceptual framework developed from previous studies guides sampling and analysis.

‡Descriptive studies are those which may be atheoretical and focus on sampling from a particular location or group.

§ Single-case studies are those which provide data from one or a very small number of participants.

NICE and SIGN guidelines can also use an adaptation of an assessment known as GRADE (Grading of Recommendations Assessment, Development and Evaluation), which is an approach to assessing the quality of evidence (NICE, 2009). Recommendations are then constructed by a review panel in which many aspects of the literature include clinical- and cost-effectiveness. The recommendations may be indicated as strong to weak, where strong recommendations are a product of a high-quality evidence base.

Criticisms of systematic reviews and meta-analyses

SRs are not without their critics, however. The eminent psychologist Eysenck (1995) outlines some criticisms in the box below.

Box 8.3:   Criticisms of systematic reviews, adapted from Eysenck (1995)

1. Including all possible studies means just that: everything – good, bad and indifferent – is included, and so the exemplary studies and their estimation of treatment effects can be corrupted by poorer work. Rather, it would be more useful to look for inconsistencies and anomalies in the data.

(Continued)

(Continued)

2. Meta-analyses give simplified answers that do not take into account the interplay of multiple variables and reducing the coverage of material included in reviews makes it difficult to consider explanations which do not appear in the included studies.
3. Meta-analysis is only meaningful if there is a high degree of homogeneity, that is, if the studies are relatively similar, and if they are relatively dissimilar (heterogeneous) their combination is difficult, if not meaningless.

Eysenck (1995, page 73) concludes by saying that if a medical treatment had an effect so recondite (difficult to understand) and obscure as to require meta-analysis to establish it, he would not be happy to have it used on him. However, it is fair to say that the science of meta-analysis has moved on considerably since he wrote this, and evidence-based or informed decision making is now established as a global strategy for improving healthcare practice.

Critiquing a systematic review and meta-analysis

Although SRs published by Cochrane are likely to be exhaustive and authoritative, not all SRs in all journals will be as good. It is possible that you may find considerably poorer ones. Hemingway and Brereton (2009) list the following as essential issues in ascertaining the quality of an SR and meta-analysis paper:

1. Is the topic well defined? Is there a clear and clinically relevant question which the reviewers seek to answer?
2. Was the search for papers thorough?
3. Were the criteria for inclusion applied fairly and consistently?
4. Was quality assessed independently by reviewers?
5. Was any missing information sought from authors?
6. Do the included studies indicate similar effects? If not, has heterogeneity been assessed?
7. Are the overall findings robust? Has publication bias been addressed?
8. Has the impact of chance been addressed? If there are few studies with statistically significant findings, does that indicate flaws in the studies, or gaps in the literature, or is there really nothing known about the question?
9. Are the recommendations clearly based on the evidence from the review? Or has any element of bias been introduced by reviewers?

CASP provides a tool for critiquing SRs and meta-analyses, and students should use this in the same way as has been discussed previously: read through the SR paper you are interested in and, using the CASP tool, make notes and look up key concepts. Question 4 asks:

Did the review's authors do enough to assess quality of the included studies?

The hint is … the authors need to consider the rigour of the studies they have identified. Lack of rigour may affect the studies' results ('All that glisters is not gold', *The Merchant of Venice* – Act II Scene 7). This is an indication of the importance of quality assessment, as discussed above. What methods of quality assurance have been used? What frameworks have they used? Has this been undertaken, discussed and agreed between members of a team rather than one author alone? Is all of this transparent?

The issue with Cochrane, Joanna Briggs Institute and other systematic reviews published in better journals is that they will be excellent, authoritative, thorough, scientific and impressive pieces of work, and this holds regardless of whether they are quantitative with statistical meta-analysis or qualitative with narrative synthesis. Therefore, you may not find faults to criticise, but critical appraisal does not necessarily mean fault finding; it can be that the studies are in fact excellent. In that case, for your assignments you will need to show that you understand the theories behind them and why they are so good.

Chapter summary

In this chapter, we began by outlining the rationale for SRs and meta-analyses. This was that there are vast quantities of research evidence available, and techniques have been developed to synthesise these so that results from many studies can be viewed as a whole to provide useful overviews for healthcare decision making. We then looked at how to construct a protocol for an SR and meta-analysis, making the point that these include thorough and exhaustive literature searching and appraisal of the evidence. Next, we introduced relevant quantitative and qualitative techniques used in meta-analysis, before moving on to talk about the Cochrane Collaboration, and how SRs and meta-analyses inform the production of clinical guidelines and the work of NICE and SIGN. Also, we have shown how to use the CASP tool to critically appraise a SR review.

Further reading

Britten, N, Campbell, R, Pope, C, Donovan, J, Morgan, M and Pill, R (2002) Using meta-ethnography to synthesise qualitative research: a worked example. *Journal of Health Services Research and Policy*, 7 (4): 209–15.

Some further insights into using meta-ethnography to synthesise qualitative research.

Crombie, IK and Davies, HTO (2009) *What Is Meta Analysis?* (2nd edition). Available online at www.betterevaluation.org/sites/default/files/Meta-An.pdf.

This is particularly relevant to issues in this chapter.

Garside, R, Britten, N and Stein, K (2008) The experience of heavy menstrual bleeding: a systematic review and meta-ethnography of qualitative studies. *Journal of Advanced Nursing*, 63 (6): 550–62.

An example of a qualitative systematic review.

Gough, D, Oliver, S and Thomas, J (2017) *An Introduction to Systematic Reviews* (2nd edition). London: Sage.

A good introduction by authors from the EPPI-Centre for Systematic Reviews (see Useful websites, below).

Greenhalgh, T (1997) How to read a paper: papers that summarise other papers (systematic reviews and meta-analyses). *British Medical Journal*, 315: 672–75.

Classic paper on this area.

Heyvaert, M, Maes, B and Onghena, P (2013) Mixed methods research synthesis: definition, framework, and potential. *Quality & Quantity*, 47 (2): 659–76.

Higgins, JTP, Thompson, SG, Deeks, JJ and Altman, DG (2003) Measuring inconsistency in meta-analyses. *British Medical Journal*, 327 (7414): 557–60. Available online at www.ncbi.nlm.nih.gov/pubmed/12958120.

Sandelowski, M and Barroso, J (2007) *Handbook for Synthesising Qualitative Research*. New York: Springer.

Souza, JP, Pileggi, C and Cecatti, JG (2007) Assessment of funnel plot asymmetry and publication bias in reproductive health meta-analyses: an analytic survey. *Reproductive Health*, 4: 3.

This study looks at publication bias in systematic reviews and meta-analyses in reproductive research.

Webb, C and Roe, B (2006) *Reviewing Research Evidence for Nursing Practice: Systematic Reviews*. Oxford: Blackwell.

Lots of good examples of qualitative systematic reviews.

Useful websites

http://eppi.ioe.ac.uk/cms

The Evidence for Policy and Practice Information and Co-ordinating Centre (EPPI-Centre) is part of the Social Science Research Unit at the Institute of Education, University of London. They conduct systematic reviews and develop methodological aspects.

www.prisma-statement.org

PRISMA (Preferred Reporting Items for Systematic Reviews and Meta-Analyses) provides an evidence-based minimum set of items for reporting in systematic reviews and meta-analyses.

http://medicine.exeter.ac.uk/esmi/workstreams/pensr

PenSR is the Peninsula Systematic Review discussion group. This is part of a South West collaborative partnership between the NHS and academia concerning evidence synthesis and involvement in research that reflects real clinical concern. This website contains useful seminar materials.

Translating evidence into practice

Chapter aims

After reading this chapter, you should be able to:

- understand the importance of evidence-informed decision making;
- understand issues and barriers involved in translating evidence into practice;
- be familiar with some of the key processes and frameworks that can aid evidence-informed decision making, and some of the influential organisations that are active in this area;
- have a working knowledge of methods for improving services.

Introduction

In this chapter we are going to discuss several things: we will begin by outlining the importance of evidence-informed decision making (EIDM). Although definitions vary, central features in the use of best evidence are: asking clinical questions, searching for and appraising relevant literature, aggregating this literature and deciding whether it is of sufficient quality and strength to be important, and using it with patients and clients. We have examined some aspects of this already in this book, and we now move on to examine how evidence can be implemented. There is a strong argument that healthcare research and evidence do not mean much unless they contribute to clinical care (or decision making). However, there are a number of issues and barriers involved in translating evidence into practice, and it is important to understand these as challenges that can be overcome. There are some key processes and frameworks that can aid EIDM, and some influential organisations that are active in this area. Lastly, we will look at concepts of service improvement.

The importance of evidence-based decision making

Evidence-based decision making has a long history in world healthcare practice and you will see it given many titles, including evidence-based medicine and nursing, and evidence-based practice (EBP). Indeed, the concept of using an evidence base to inform decision making is now widespread and used in many sectors, from healthcare to social work and even forestry. Evidence-based practice (EBP) was initially hailed as a new way of delivering (medical) care, which would overturn the 'unscientific' features of intuition and unsystematic clinical experience and, instead, provide a systematic rationale for clinical decision making based on evidence from clinical research (Guyatt, 1991). Since then, what is effectively a whole new science has evolved, concerning evidence, its synthesis and its clinical implementation.

A couple of very famous and oft-repeated quotes illustrate this. EIDM is

> *the conscientious, explicit, and judicious use of current best evidence in making decisions about the care of individual patients. The practice of evidence-based medicine means integrating individual clinical expertise with the best available external clinical evidence from systematic research.*

> (Sackett et al., 1996, page 312)

Others have subsequently emphasised the importance of including concepts of patient-centredness, so that decisions about treatments are made in conjunction with the patient and the clinician. Therefore, EIDM is

> *an approach to decision making in which the clinician uses the best evidence available, in consultation with the patient, to decide upon the option which suits the patient best.*

> (Muir Gray, 2009)

This latter definition has a focus on what works best for individual patients, therefore indicating the need to translate research (that often takes place in idealised conditions) into workable and effective treatments for individuals, groups and populations of people in the real world.

Translating research into practice

Regardless of the quality of research, a consistent failure in clinical and health services research is the inability of researchers to translate their evidence into practice and policy developments that actually benefit patients and healthcare, and this is an international problem that has been the subject of increasing attention recently. The literature draws a distinction between T1 research (the translation of basic biomedical research into clinical science and knowledge) and T2 research (the translation of new knowledge into improved care). It is this latter aspect, implementing new knowledge and translating evidence into developing healthcare practice, that is most important for nurses and patients (Grimshaw et al., 2012).

McGlynn et al. (2003) estimate that, overall, Americans only receive about half of the care and treatments that their conditions require, meaning, for example, that people with diabetes do not receive adequate blood glucose monitoring, elderly people do not receive flu vaccines and blood pressure is not appropriately monitored. Those with alcohol dependence seem to fare worst, receiving only 10 per cent of their recommended care. All of these examples stem from the failure to implement evidence and clinical guidelines, and they have measureable impacts on morbidity and mortality for patients and incur costs to the healthcare system.

Research summary 9.1: Evidence-informed decision making

There are many examples of how EIDM has positively impacted on clinical practice.

- Greenhalgh (2014) quotes the British Thoracic Society's 1990 asthma guidelines (updated and revised regularly since 1990, including in 2019), based on randomised trials and observational studies, which helped establish correct prescribing and self-management plans, to substantially reduce asthma morbidity and mortality.
- The Cochrane Collaboration logo (see Chapter 8, page 155 incorporates a forest plot from a particular EIDM study: the meta-analysis of the use of corticosteroids with pregnant women to improve outcomes for their premature babies whose lungs had failed to develop sufficiently before birth. Without steroids, the resulting infant respiratory distress syndrome causes early death and permanent disability. The initial science relating to corticosteroid usage in lambs began in 1969, with human studies first undertaken in the 1970s, but this was not translated into widespread practice until decades later. Crowley and others worked on literature reviews in the 1980s which were first published as a systematic review in 1989 (Roberts and Dalziel, 2006).

Using evidence can be crucial in developing and changing practice, and evidence will continually evolve, so in that sense EIDM is aspirational: we must carry on using the best available evidence, understanding that that evidence may change in quality, emphasis and impact. In recognition of the importance of translating research findings into developments in clinical practice the current NHS constitution gives a commitment to innovate and to use research to improve health and care (Department of Health, 2015 and updated in 2023).

Issues and barriers to evidence-informed decision making

If there is consensus that healthcare could do better at translating research into practice, why does this not occur and/or not occur in a more timely fashion? Modifying practice and clinicians' behaviour is complex, multidimensional, and difficult, but not impossible. Strategies to promote EIDM that overcome these issues are required and simply exhorting individuals to do better will not work. Indeed, there is a strong argument that solutions must be tailored to different settings, patient groups and practitioners (Grol and Grimshaw, 2003). Two types of EIDM are prevalent in healthcare organisations: engaging in EIDM activities such as searching for and critically appraising evidence for practice, and using evidence including guidelines, protocols and care pathways for changing nursing practice (Yost et al., 2014). Research indicates that, while nurses and midwives are well aware of the importance of evidence for practice, their knowledge about exactly what it means and how to go about implementing it is much less substantial (Melnyk et al., 2004), and that trying to implement protocols and guidelines is frequently problematic (Grol and Grimshaw, 2003).

It seems as if the key issues that prevent the implementation of evidence in nursing practice are limited resources, lack of time and resistance to change. Conversely, things that facilitate EIDM are organisational drivers including prioritisation, resource allocation and creating an effective evidence culture, with tools to support and facilitate staff to make research-based changes. Multifaceted strategies are required, and many such projects include an educational component, but other examples exist indicating that some progress can be made with single interventions such as audit and feedback, clinical decision support systems, local opinion leaders, library access, journal clubs, evidence-based training, team-learning activities, activities conducted by nurse managers, external inspection and appreciative inquiry (Ellen et al., 2014). However, it is likely that implementation and knowledge translation depend on targeted interventions for different audiences, recent and relevant systematic reviews or other syntheses of research findings and awareness of the local context in terms of the clinical setting and personnel, informed by an assessment of the likely barriers and facilitators (Grimshaw et al., 2012). What is also important is having an element of leadership or change agency and, as part of this, key features are the characteristics of a leader in clinical practice, their interaction with others in the organisation and the context in which the care takes place. Successful change is likely to need an accessible change agent who is compatible with the local culture, who models behaviour and who enables reflection on practice (McCormack et al., 2013).

Activity 9.1 Evidence-based practice

Think about the clinical care that you are involved with. Ask your supervisors in clinical practice about some aspect of care or a procedure that you are interested in. Ask them if they know of policy or guidelines, research or other types of evidence that supports doing 'it' (whatever 'it' is) in the way that they do it. Go home and do a very quick literature search, perhaps using your university library databases, then the NICE and Cochrane databases. Have a brief read of what comes up and summarise the following:

1. Does the evidence you have found broadly support or contradict what is happening in practice?
2. What types of evidence have you found? Is it primary research (a single empirical study)? Is it secondary like NICE guidance or systematic reviews?
3. If you are able, discuss your findings with your practice supervisor and try to find out between you what you think are the issues and barriers if that clinical area wanted to implement some new practice. Be sensitive about this please so it is not perceived as criticism.

As this is a personal research exercise, there is no answer at the end of the chapter.

Frameworks for implementation

Many authors have grappled with the complexity of how best to translate research findings into practical applications in real-world healthcare. We will now briefly discuss three of the better-known ones, these being the PARiHS (Promoting Action on Research Implementation in Health Services) framework (Kitson et al., 1998; Kitson et al., 2008), the Knowledge to Action framework (KtA) (Graham et al., 2006), and the Joanna Briggs Institute Model of Evidence-Based Health Care (JBI EBHC). All three attempt to synthesise literature about how best to use evidence in practice and their findings illustrate and guide a detailed analysis of the nature of evidence, context and personnel to enable changes in care.

Promoting action on research implementation in a health services' framework

The PARiHS framework (Kitson et al., 1998; Kitson et al., 2008) incorporates themes from the literature on implementation including:

- organisational rather than individual responsibilities;
- that research evidence must be strong (for example, systematic reviews or clinical guidelines) before implementation is justified;
- the need for careful planning and a range of interventions.

Kitson and colleagues also recommend that criteria for evaluating the impact of the intervention must be identified before the process starts. PARiHS can be used to guide research implementation, with three key elements identified as important: evidence, context and facilitation, each of which has sub-elements that can be rated on a scale from low to high. High ratings on each factor are more likely to produce successful implementation of research results (Kitson et al., 1998; Kitson et al., 2008; National Collaborating Centre for Methods and Tools, 2011). Broadly conceptualised (see Figure 9.1), it is the function of facilitation (or 'leadership' or 'change agency') to drive implementation into the upper right quadrant, which shows the ideal situation for implementing research in practice. PARiHS offers a useful diagnostic framework but success may not always be possible if the research evidence is weak or non-existent.

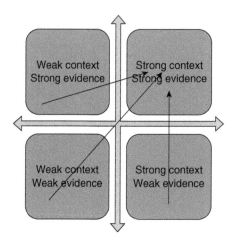

Figure 9.1 The PARiHS Diagnostic and Evaluative Grid (adapted from original material by Kitson et al. 2008, published in an Open Access article distributed under the terms of the Creative Commons Attribution License which permits unrestricted use, distribution, and reproduction in any medium, provided the original work is properly cited)

Knowledge to action (KtA) framework

This framework was developed as a response to the apparent confusion about numerous concepts relating to getting evidence into practice, and Graham et al. (2006) analyse these ideas and offer a conceptual framework as a guideline for integrating the roles of knowledge creation and knowledge application. They divided these two activities so that knowledge creation appears as a 'funnel' shape indicating the increasing 'usefulness' of evidence for practice which comes from knowledge synthesis in the form of systematic reviews and meta-analysis and guidelines. These aggregate related studies, which can be refined to produce highly relevant clinical decision-making tools to guide practice, meaning that clinicians can answer the question 'what works best?' The knowledge application element is shown as an action cycle, with a series of stages that will aid implementation of evidence. These stages require planning and design to make sure that the evidence, education, context and personnel are aligned, so that knowledge utilisation is effective and sustainable so that clinicians can answer the question 'how should we implement the evidence?' It may be necessary to adapt national guidelines to a local clinical context in order to make them more relevant and directly applicable (Harrison et al., 2010).

Joanna Briggs Institute model of evidence-based health care

The Joanna Briggs Institute (JBI) has emerged as a major international force in evidence synthesis, implementation science and facilitation of evidence-based healthcare. They argue that lasting change in health systems needs multi-level activity to identify barriers and enablers to evidence-based health care (EBHC), with four overarching factors to be considered; these being culture, capacity, communication and collaboration. All of these factors would need consideration within healthcare systems if sustainable, evidence-informed change is to be generated. Their model also emphasises that evidence-informed decision-making needs to take into account whether or not research on interventions and treatments have feasibility, acceptability, meaningfulness and effectiveness (FAME) (Jordan et al., 2016). JBI FAME has a detailed handbook regarding evidence implementation available via their website (**https://jbi-global-wiki. refined.site/space/JHEI**) and an interesting interactive model, which puts patients and decision makers at its centre.

Activity 9.2   Using the JBI FAME model to consider how evidence might inform clinical decision making

Watch this video about how the JBI FAME model works and puts patients at the heart of clinical decision making **https://youtu.be/zO4J8o-6Krs?si=lMEniHta7XeD9nhV**

You can access the JBI FAME model here **https://jbi.global/jbi-model-of-EBHC**.

When you are reading research papers for your own purposes you can think through whether in your opinion their results meet the JBI FAME criteria; that is, are they:

- feasible;
- acceptable;
- meaningful;
- effective.

There is a worked example based on a research study by Liao et al. (2018) at the end of the chapter.

Improving quality for better patient care
We'll now turn to the concept of quality improvement importance, concepts and relevance

Life in organisations never stands still and the NHS is no different. Historically the concept of continuous quality improvement was imported from industry where free-market competition and new consumer demands, production techniques and technological advancement have meant that, in order to survive, firms must innovate, improving quality and developing the range of products that they sell. These developments have been applied to healthcare organisations around the world as, to borrow a phrase from industry, the marketplace for care and the demands of our 'customers' are changing: technological improvements, an ageing population and a focus on improving the patient experience all require attention from nurses working in an environment characterised by budgetary constraints. So much so that many authors believe that service improvement now needs to be an integral part of all nurses' approach to the care they deliver (Smith et al., 2014).

In a general sense, it is useful to think about improving services as being

> *a planned and targeted effort to improve patient-facing outcomes from a service, whether process outcomes, such as throughput; or final outcomes, such as treatment. Service improvement is thus a useful intermediate measure of performance in a service organization. Service improvement may both create and reduce costs, as well as improving clinical outcomes.*

(Fitzgerald et al., 2013)

We have seen from the discussions above that there is now a major focus on translating research into practice, and this can be considered service improvement in the most generic sense. Service improvement may not necessarily be evidence-based, but nowadays NHS Trusts would require service improvement activities to take evidence into account and might demand evidence-based rationales as part of their clinical governance approval processes. These types of activities may be termed 'clinical effectiveness' in some NHS Trust governance structures. Where there are new or updated NICE guidelines, these may need to be explicitly integrated into clinical care activities, and the evidence base and the assessment of its strength would be part of the NICE guideline.

We have also discussed the concept of 'facilitation' above in relation to evidence implementation in practice. This is an important concept in service improvement and is more commonly termed leadership. Leadership development focused on local service development has been found to be an essential facet of driving change (Kitson et al., 2011; Fealy et al., 2015).

Quality improvement and practice development

Conceptually, authors draw distinctions between quality improvement (QI) and practice development (PD) methodologies, with the latter often described as 'emancipatory'. Quality improvement is described as having a focus on safety, effectiveness and person-centredness (Lavery, 2017), and although co-production and activity between leaders, colleagues and patients is required for change to be successful, often QI can be problem driven, with a need to do something differently in service delivery, and an external rationale for change, for example, implementation of new NICE guidance or audit data indicating poor performance on some clinical indicators. Practice development can take a more fluid approach, with an emphasis on developing workplace culture, high-quality care and a more democratic approach to change management. Practice development also shares a desire for change that benefits patients with QI, and is further characterized as technical PD (tPD) which would appear to share many similarities with QI as briefly described immediately above, and emancipatory PD (ePD), with the emancipatory element concerned with how self-reflection and self-understanding is influenced by social conditions (Manley and McCormack, 2003), and how collaboration and mutuality can be harnessed to change working conditions for the better, There is an explicit reference to the critical social sciences in ePD, meaning the analysis of power relations, and how changing them can benefit patients and staff.

Although much of the emphasis of QI and PD is superficially similar, Lavery (2017) indicates that both methodologies have difficulties in differentiating their approaches but share the concern to build an environment in which enthusiastic and expert staff work in organisations with improved processes. As we shall see below, however, despite similarities there are differences in terminology and approaches ('methodologies') between QI and PD. Although there are many different conceptualisations of QI and PD approaches, we will look at two QI approaches, and one PD approach, with case study examples for all three.

Approaches to quality improvement: PDSA

We have seen above some fairly complex frameworks for implementing evidence. There are numerous frameworks for QI, but one championed by the NHS as simple, effective and referred to by some authors (Williams and Caley, 2020), as the model for improvement is plan, do, study, act (PDSA). This seeks answers to the questions:

- What are we trying to accomplish?
- How will we know that a change is an improvement?
- What changes can we make that will result in the improvements that we seek?

It is simply drawn as a circular diagram, which can undergo much iteration, with stages overlapping or continuous (see Figure 9.2).

The idea behind PDSA is that a team involved in a service would have a preliminary idea about how that service might be developed. This could be from a variety of sources but would normally include patient satisfaction feedback, evidence in the form of guidelines, research and/or cost-effectiveness data. The team would require leadership in its goals, and would begin with a *Planning* phase, identifying exactly what needed to change, how this might be made to happen and who would be involved. An important element in this planning is likely to be process mapping. This involves examining the patient journey and finding out if there are obvious issues, bottlenecks or faults in their clinical care or its administration and processes that can be identified and rectified. It may be that complex flow diagrams are created that indicate the stages that a patient has to go through to get investigation results, diagnosis and treatment, and this may involve significant time delays and multiple returns to hospital, clinics or GP services. Once the QI team understands these processes, they can be altered to get beneficial changes for patients by, for example, using tools to ensure appropriate referrals, reducing return visits or cutting down waiting times. Part of the QI process might be to look at existing care pathways for that patient/client group's journey. NICE Quality Standards, which have been developed using best practice evidence and indicate how NICE guidance can be implemented, and even how other services are delivered more effectively in other areas. For example, the NICE Quality Standard Alcohol-use disorders: diagnosis and management (QS11, 2023) contains the following quality statement:

- Adults who are being asked about their alcohol use have a validated alcohol questionnaire completed to identify any need for a brief intervention or referral to specialist alcohol services.

This may seem obvious to use a diagnostic tool to identify the need for treatment, but if a nurse was working in an area where that was *not* usual practice, there would be a need to introduce such a tool. Such a tool would need to be evidence-based, with research indicating it was valid, reliable and effective, and would standardise referrals to specialist alcohol services, reducing variations between staff completing the assessment. This would be likely to improve care for patients if it ensured the right patients were getting the right journey and may reduce the burden on the specialist alcohol service through reducing inappropriate referrals, giving them more time to see the patients in the most need. Implementing this tool and changing service delivery and referral practices would be much more likely to be successful if it was a planned QI project, with education and team ownership, as opposed to something imposed by management without consultation and collaboration.

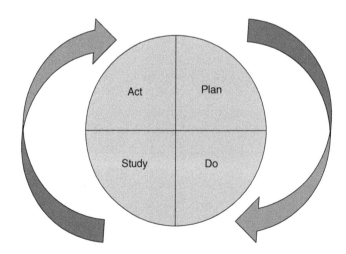

Figure 9.2 Plan, do, study, act cycles and the model for improvement (**https://aqua. nhs.uk/wp-content/uploads/2023/07/qsir-pdsa-cycles-model-for-improvement.pdf**).

The team would then *Do* the change, which is the implementation phase. The successes and challenges of this implementation phase would then be *Studied* in some formal sense: this evaluation might involve examining the newly developed service using a variety of outcome measures; in our alcohol treatment example above, it might be comparing referrals pre- and post-project. Lastly, when all the data is processed, it might be necessary to take further *Action*, meaning that the team would learn from their implementation experience, revise how they were doing things and then incorporate that learning into the new service as it becomes routine practice.

There are many examples of successful service improvement projects, from local to system level, two of which are outlined in the case studies below.

Case study 9.1: Better access for patients with breathing problems

The PDSA framework was used by one NHS Trust in response to concerns about the difficulties patients with chronic obstructive pulmonary disease were encountering in accessing emergency services (Dodds et al., 2006). The delays and frustrations experienced by these patients meant they remained in hospital longer than was necessary. A redesign of emergency access arrangements at the hospital for patients with COPD aimed to:

- decrease patient journey time;
- improve patient, carer and staff experiences; and
- reduce process variability.

Service users were actively involved in developing the changes, as their voice was heard in the focus groups that were part of the planning stage. During the project, innovative roles were implemented and evaluated, which led to improved access to the respiratory wards and specialist personnel.

Overall, there was a reduction in the average length of stay for patients (down from a ten-and-a-half day stay to six days) and an increase in the numbers of patients admitted directly to the emergency medical unit and transferred to the respiratory department, which had implications for service quality and safety for these vulnerable people with this chronic long-term condition.

Lean methodology

The lean approach originated in manufacturing at Toyota and is intended to continually focus on what customers value and remove what customers do not value (Lavery, 2017), to streamline and simplify processes and eradicate waste. There is a framework based on five features which are:

1. Understanding and identifying value. The organisation needs to engage with customers to understand what they want, need and value.

2. Mapping the value stream. This involves creating a physical map, for example a patient's journey, to see what processes look like.

3. Creating flow. How can an organisation improve all aspects of what they do?

4. Establishing pull. When does the customer need the service?

5. Seeking perfection. A constant focus on activity to increase value for customers, so that beneficial change never ceases.

Case study 9.2: Nurse-led liaison mental health service for older adults

Atkinson and Mukaetova-Ladinska (2012) discuss how Specialised Liaison Psychiatric Services for Older Adults have been established in the UK but with considerable variations in service delivery and quality across the UK, and with a problem of under-referral to the service in their NHS Trust. Using lean principles, they sought to increase referrals, reduce waiting times to be seen and increase specialist liaison nurse availability on the ward. Using a lean approach, they were quickly able to drive change and enhance processes and care in this area, with an increase in referrals from seven in two months pre-project, to 20 in the two months post-project, and the waiting times to be seen down from five days to one day. There were similarly impressive reductions in length of stay, readmissions and patients remaining out of hospital. The authors conclude their study demonstrates that some of the identified changes can be implemented promptly and within available and unchanged resources, at speed and with clear auditable outcomes.

Approaches to practice development

The approaches outlined above can have reasonably clear steps for implementation and can be structured with measurable outcomes to provide an indication that aims and objectives have been achieved. Practice development approaches seldom seem so clear-cut when reading published accounts, but this can be seen as a strength as well as a limitation: what they lack in clarity can also be seen as a flexibility that allows practitioners to focus on what is important for staff and patients rather than being solution based and about implementing externally driven evidence. One of the seminal PD authors (McCormack et al, 2013) indicates that there is a high degree of methodological diversity in published work, but also that key features of PD are a desire to foster person-centred care, collaboration and partnership, facilitation and support, active learning and development, transforming workplace cultures, and evaluation.

For many authors, two crucial elements in operationalising PD methodology are the concepts of facilitation and critical reflection. As the theoretical antecedents of PD are critical social theory, with a focus on power relations, PD authors emphasise how facilitators should work with staff with the goal of enhancing patient care, safety and valuing the individual patient and groups of staff. Facilitation is powerful and can take many forms; for example, Hardiman and Dewing (2019) argue that facilitation of practice development and workplace learning are effective methods to develop person-centred cultures and use the concept of 'critical companionship' in their work. Expert facilitation for person-centred cultures is described as creating an effective workplace culture in wich everyone can flourish, and/or create 'good places to work' (Middleton et al., 2021). How this is to be achieved is described in multiple different ways by authors, for example Cook (2023) champions clinical supervision, McCance and McCormack (2021) discuss the need for critical reflection and 'knowing self', and latterly McCormack (2021) champions working on the core aspects of our being including values and beliefs, which can be transformed to the benefit of patient-centred healthcare.

Case study 9.3: Using electronic records to foster compassionate care in an acute hospital in Ireland

Hardiman et al. (2020) discuss how they introduced an updated and enhanced electronic record system, and they sought to make it holistic, involve all stakeholders, and show evidence of person-centred nursing practice. A team including facilitator, assistant director of nursing and a nurse IT specialist spent three days exploring the vision and values of nursing documentation to make sure they reflected personal and organisational values. This enabled them to develop a shared vision including evidence-based care and incorporate international nursing language into their record keeping. To ensure participation in the process, cycles of repeated activity were implemented to include all the stakeholders. Overall, they conclude that the project was successful because of widespread stakeholder involvement, which ensured the external company providing the IT upgrade acted in accordance with the values and needs of the system users. Using PD methodology, the team implemented a record that would support and enhance the relationship between nurses and patients, as one element of a wider transformation of organisational culture at their hospital.

Activity 9.3   Evidence-based practice

Ask your supervisors in clinical practice about any recent changes in service delivery or processes that have occurred recently. In particular, ask them:

1.   How and why have things changed?
2.   What was the evidence for the change?
3.   Who led the changes and how did they involve staff?
4.   How has the change been evaluated? What data have you seen relating to the change?

As this is a personal research exercise there is no answer at the end of the chapter.

Activity 9.4   Using JBI FAME to consider evidence for practice

Find and read this research study: Liao et al. (2018).

Using the JBI FAME concept can help you to analyse this paper and reflect on how the results might be useful inpatient care. When you are doing this, you will be thinking through how this research study might inform clinical decision making: you are using a model of EHBC, thinking about if the research is clinically effective or not, and engaging in evidence-informed decision making as a result.

The authors indicate that China has the highest prevalence of cigarette smokers, accounting for more than 40 per cent of the total cigarette consumption in the world, but as smoking cessation services were limited in China at the time of the study, the authors wanted to assess if text messaging might help people to quit. In an RCT comparing high frequency, low frequency and control text messaging (the control messages were not about stopping smoking), people in the high frequency group were most likely to stop, but those in the low frequency group stopped nearly as much, when compared to the group who got unrelated control texts. Liao et al. (2018) conclude that their intervention works and might be useful to others designing smoking cessation services.

- Think of JBI FAME. What comments would you make about feasibility, acceptability, meaningfulness and effectiveness?
- Thinking about a patient you cared for, how could the result have influenced the care given by the MDT?
- Can you find any particular strengths and weaknesses with the paper?

Below in Table 9.1 are some brief notes which allow you to use JBI FAME to analyse this paper and reflect on how it might influence patient care.

Action research

Action research (AR) relates to a broad category of research designs that attempt to change some aspect of social life, and it has been used in myriad settings across the globe and for many years. It can be problematic trying to show how AR is different from service development ideas. However, a simple answer would be that, while service development is primarily about developing the service in question, AR would be about developing the service as well as learning about the experience (through researching it). Coghlan and Brannick (2019) discuss how AR has several key characteristics, including being about research in action rather than just about the action, and so 'scientific' processes of inquiry are important to demonstrate rigour in data collection and analysis. Participants are involved in experiencing some issue that requires change, developing solutions and studying the change processes they instigate. AR, more explicitly perhaps than service development models, is a collaborative, democratic process and, while we have discussed process mapping and care pathways above, most AR

Table 9.1   Using JBI FAME to analyse and reflect

JBI FAME?	MDT patient care	Strengths and weaknesses
Feasible? Seems very feasible to send text messages, even to a very large population like in China. Acceptable? The study indicates that it is acceptable and would appear so assuming motivation to quit smoking. Meaningful? Seemed to make a difference to smoking rates. Effective? The paper indicates that it should work, and although not tested, would be highly cost effective too.	Imagine you have a patient with COPD, asthma or lung cancer, or a patient with severe mental health issues, or a pregnant woman who wanted to stop for her baby. If this service was available in your area, would you refer that person on to this service? How might this have changed the care they received from you? Think about the health benefits and financial cost savings that person would make.	Strengths Large sample in China. Virtually everyone has a mobile phone. Objective measurement of quitting. Weaknesses Participants were able to use other smoking cessation services as well (doesn't say this in the abstract but it's there in the full paper), so can't be sure if the texts made the difference of not. This seems like quite a major flaw. We know however that at the time of the study there was little smoking cessation available in China so it is a judgement about just how effective this study may be.

would not have an external agenda in the way that might happen if adopting a care pathway or NICE guidance. Indeed, AR would value more highly the active participation of those involved, whether patients, staff or collaborations between the two groups. This is distinct from traditional research approaches, both quantitative and qualitative, where research participants are subjects rather than collaborators, but in AR there is always some spiral design process (similar to the PDSA module in Figure 9.2) so that change occurs while knowledge is generated (Williamson et al., 2012).

AR has received some focus in the NHS but seems to have been superseded more recently by the service development ideas we have discussed above. For example, Waterman et al. (2001) were commissioned by the NHS Health Technology Assessment programme to examine AR's potential as a localised change management strategy. However, a search on the NHS England website in 2024 identified only one example of AR and several thousand examples of service or quality improvement projects. This may, in part, be due to the tension between action researchers traditionally insisting on imprecision in defining their field, when the NHS wants defined strategies and outcomes, particularly where there is a need to implement NICE guidelines or streamline service delivery to optimise patient outcomes such as timely referrals or more effective triage There may also be some wariness because some AR can be explicitly political. This does not mean that AR cannot be used for service development or beneficial change in clinical care. Indeed, there are many global examples of clinical and organisation change in the AR literature (Williamson et al., 2012). It is only that the NHS has perhaps moved on in the production of harder measures like process mapping and care pathways.

Chapter summary

In this chapter we have examined a number of issues concerning translating research into practice. We have briefly highlighted the importance of the concept of evidence-informed decision making (EIDM) as a guide for clinical practice. It is clear that there are many issues and barriers to EIDM, and also that using frameworks for implementation including PARiHS, KtA and JBI EBHC can help practitioners to structure change in clinical practice based on evidence.

In addition, we have discussed some key recent ideas relating to the UK NHS concerning how to improve services for patients, with a focus on QI and PD frameworks.

Further reading

Kitson, A, Rycroft-Malone, J, Harvey, G, McCormack, B, Seers, K and Titchen, A (2008) Evaluating the successful implementation of evidence into practice using the PARIHS framework: theoretical and practical challenges. *Implementation Science*, 3, 1, doi:10.1186/1748-5908-3-1.

Seminal paper in this field.

Williamson, GR, Bellman, L and Webster, J (2012) *Action Research in Nursing and Healthcare.* London, Sage.

Comprehensive discussion of issues in the field of action research for practitioners.

Useful websites

www.nursingtimes.net/behind-the-rituals-blog/14137.subject

The Behind the Rituals blog in the *Nursing Times*. Explores some questions about evidence and nursing practice.

www.cebm.ox.ac.uk/

The Centre for Evidence-Based Medicine is a not-for-profit organisation dedicated to the practice, teaching and dissemination of high-quality evidence-based medicine to improve healthcare in everyday clinical practice.

www.england.nhs.uk/improvement-hub/wp-content/uploads/sites/44/2017/11/ILG-1.2-Process-Mapping-Analysis-and-Redesign.pdf

NHS Institute for Innovation and Implementation process mapping resources.

The KT Clearinghouse website is funded by the Canadian Institute of Health Research (CIHR) to serve as the repository of knowledge translation resources and provides extensive resources.

www.nice.org.uk/standards-and-indicators/how-to-use-quality-standards

How to use the NICE Quality Standards. In this page see also the link to an Excel template for service improvement and a link to the Into Practice guide.

www.health.org.uk/sites/default/files/QualityImprovementMadeSimple.pdf

The Health foundation. Quality improvement made simple. What everyone should know about healthcare quality improvement.

www.england.nhs.uk/improvement-hub/wp-content/uploads/sites/44/2017/11/Going-Lean-in-the-NHS.pdf

Going lean in the NHS.

Section 4

Writing and finishing

Chapter 10 Writing up your literature review

Chapter aims

After reading this chapter, you should be able to:

- understand the different structures that can be used for a literature review;
- structure and write up your literature review;
- organise your references in a systematic manner.

Introduction

Section 4 includes two chapters focusing on the final stage of writing up. In this chapter, we guide you through the process of structuring and writing up your literature review. This will include understanding the purpose of your literature review, identifying the different structures that can be used and appreciating the importance of being thorough and systematic.

In Chapter 11, we will introduce you to some basic writing skills and give you some tips about how to structure and write your research proposal or dissertation. We will examine what barriers you may experience to the writing process, and we will stress the importance of writing as soon as possible rather than waiting until the later stages of your project.

Writing up your literature review

In this chapter, we outline how to write up your literature review, either as a stand-alone piece of work or as part of an empirical research study. This builds upon Chapter 2, where you were introduced to the process of undertaking a literature search to identify the key literature for your research topic.

Your literature review needs to be thorough and systematic to ensure that it does not cover only the literature that supports your beliefs and therefore ignores any material that may challenge them. Indeed, the literature that challenges your beliefs can be your most valuable resource because it makes you question and explore your viewpoint.

There are a number of key elements to a literature review and the emphasis that you give to each component depends upon your individual project. The key elements are:

- definitions for the key terminology you will use;
- the historical background to your research topic and the current context of your research topic, demonstrating how it is important and relevant;
- a discussion of relevant concepts and theories that you will use;
- a critical evaluation of previous studies, addressing their strengths and weaknesses and any gaps that have not been addressed;
- if you are undertaking empirical data collection, it also enables you to justify how your research will extend or challenge previous studies or respond to a gap in your field.

Your literature review should provide a coherent and critical account of the literature, identifying patterns and themes as well as evaluating the quality of the material. One of the features of a good literature review is that it acknowledges that most topics are contested terrain in which competing viewpoints are expressed. This means that you need to provide an active account that evaluates the available evidence and demonstrates your own voice as an author, rather than a passive description of these different accounts.

Case study 10.1: Developing the structure of your literature review

Folashade is training to be a health visitor and she is interested in the role of culture in child protection. She is writing up her literature review and has written the following paragraph:

> *Qiao et al. (2018) found that culture is a powerful influence on how child abuse is understood and responded to in mainland China. Briggs and Whittaker (2018) argue that cultural contexts are very important in the protection of children from abuse within specific communities, such as child abuse linked to beliefs in witchcraft and spirit possession. Wills et al. (2017) found that culture needed a great emphasis in government initiatives. Evans and Whittaker (2010) argue that culture is not only related to race and ethnicity but can include other forms of culture, such as Deaf culture.*

Activity 10.1   Critical thinking

What are the weaknesses in this paragraph? What improvements might you recommend to Folashade?

There is a brief summary of answers and a suggested alternative paragraph at the end of the chapter.

The key message is that you need to avoid a 'shopping list' approach, in which you provide an inventory of previous research studies without an overall narrative. As well as evaluating the quality of individual studies, your analysis should make links between studies, highlighting similarities and differences and drawing out the main issues.

A good literature review will not take what has previously been written at face value but will be aware of the contested nature of knowledge, in which alternative views and positions may be taken. It will also be sensitive to issues of power, where some viewpoints are privileged while others are marginalised.

Structuring your literature review

You need to have a clear overall structure to your literature review and there are a number of different options. One option is a chronological structure, looking at how your research topic has been written about over a period of time. This is particularly useful when your research topic shows a clear historical development. For example, a literature review of patient involvement could use a specific time period and discuss how public attitudes towards health services have developed from a paternalistic model to expectations that patients are more involved in decisions about their care. Another alternative is to structure your literature review thematically, focusing on what concepts or theoretical models are addressed. Using the same example, the literature review could be structured according to the different philosophies that underpin patient involvement (managerialist versus emancipatory models) or the sites of involvement (staff recruitment, service planning and training).

A general concept used to describe the structure of literature reviews is *funnelling*. This describes a process in which the literature review begins with a broad discussion that aims to provide a backdrop or background context for the research and there is a progressive narrowing of the focus. This can be achieved in a number of ways and some commonly used structures are as follows:

- Moving from the most general literature to that which is most closely related to your work. For example, briefly discussing the wider literature in your field, focusing more on some of the literature in your general topic area but saving your most detailed analysis for the research that is closest to your research topic.
- A chronological structure, moving from the earliest literature to the most recent.
- A 'compare and contrast' or dialectical approach, in which you outline one approach, contrast it with a second approach and then introduce a third approach.

When you are preparing the outline of your literature review, it can be helpful to write a detailed argument structure. This is the series of steps that you will follow in developing your argument and enables you to establish quickly whether it has a logical progression. For example, if you were writing a literature review about bereavement using a chronological structure, your argument structure might look something like this:

1. Introduction to the concept of bereavement, including definitions.

2. Chronological review of bereavement models, such as Kübler-Ross (1993) and her stage model.

3. Critical appraisal of Kübler-Ross's model (e.g. seen as overly prescriptive with insufficient weight given to social context).

4. Discussion of more recent models of bereavement and how they address shortcomings of earlier models; for example, Walter's (1996) 'new model of grief', which focuses on sociological concepts of identity and argues that the purpose of grief is to sustain the link with the lost person rather than to 'move on'.

5. Conclusion – review of developments in models of bereavement.

Try to avoid overly relying upon headings to communicate your structure to the reader. Indeed, it is worth checking with your supervisor because some universities discourage the use of headings and subheadings, while other assignments require a clear structure and headings. You should include 'signposting' statements at key points to help the reader understand what has been discussed and what you are moving on to; for example, 'Having defined partnership working, the next step is to discuss how each agency has a different role'. These are statements that indicate a transition between sections by reminding the reader of what has already been discussed and indicating what will be discussed next.

Literature reviews in empirical studies

If you are collecting your own data, your literature review needs to make an argument for your proposed research. In particular, it needs to directly address your research question and how you intend to respond to it. Aveyard (2023) makes the useful suggestion to insert your research question in the header and footer section of your document to ensure that you maintain your focus. Do not be tempted to extend out to issues that are interesting but outside your research question. Rather than a wide-ranging discussion of all the topics that could be relevant to your study, you should aim to produce a focused piece of work that makes the argument for your proposed study. This will often include gaps in the previous literature or methodological innovations that you would like to introduce.

Designing your research study will require you to make active choices and you need to show how these decisions were informed by your literature review. So, as well as the literature on your topic, you need to discuss the methodological literature. Whether this is included in your literature review, or your methodology section will depend upon your individual research project and the approach of your university, so it is advisable to check this out with your supervisor.

A note on terminology

There are a number of common confusions in terminology that relate to how you use referencing in your literature review:

- Reference list versus bibliography: a common confusion is between a reference list and a bibliography; these are often used as if they are interchangeable terms. A reference list includes only those texts that you have cited in the main body of your literature. A bibliography includes all the texts that you have read while preparing your literature review, whether or not you have cited them. You will always need to provide a reference list, but you are not always required to provide a bibliography. Indeed, if your university uses one of the more popular referencing systems such as the Harvard system (i.e. author name and date in text), a bibliography is not normally required.

- Citation versus references: another potential source of confusion is between a citation and a reference. The term 'citation' refers to the text within the main body of your literature review that informs the reader of which texts you are drawing upon. Strictly speaking, references refer to the systematic list of texts at the end of your literature review that includes all of the texts that you have cited, but it is often used informally as synonymous with a citation.

- Footnotes versus endnotes: footnotes and endnotes are usually in the form of numbered entries embedded in the main part of the text which direct the reader to a separate note at the foot of the page (footnotes) or a separate list at the end of the document (endnotes). They have traditionally been used for additional material, such as comments, thoughts and anecdotes that were not considered important enough to include in the main body of the text.

Using reference management software

There are a number of software packages available to help you manage your references. Current examples include Mendeley, EndNote, RefWorks, Papers and CiteULike. These are constantly developing, and web-based versions have been developed using cloud technology that enables you to use the software from any computer.

Reference management software generally works as a database, collecting together the references for all the material that you are using to write your literature review. They link with word-processing software such as Microsoft Word, enabling you to insert citations in the main body of your text and automatically generate a reference list at the end of your text. This reduces the risk of one of the most frequent problems with academic coursework, namely, inaccurate reference lists. It is common for lecturers to mark work that has a reference list that does not include all of the material cited but instead includes additional material that the student intended to use but never got round to including.

Another advantage of reference management software is that some of the texts are likely to be used in other academic work so the material can be reused. Ideally, students should learn to use reference management software at the beginning of their studies to gain maximum benefit, but final-year students can get immediate benefits and hopefully will return for further study.

Some packages offer additional features. For example, Mendeley enables the user to store articles in a similar way to the music management software iTunes. When articles are imported in PDF format, the software automatically recognises key information (journal title, year, author, title and so on) and the article can be tagged and arranged into bibliographies or 'playlists' for different projects. Articles can be shared with other users, who can be invited to view specific material or the whole database of articles. When choosing reference management software, it is worth checking out these additional features.

Some common challenges when writing a literature review

There are a number of challenges that students can experience while completing their literature reviews.

How do I decide what to include and what to leave out?

One of the most common problems with literature reviews is that students try to use every piece of material that they have read. This is at least partly because considerable work has gone into identifying and reading the material and the student wants the marker to know this. Although it can be disheartening to leave out material that you have worked hard on, it is almost essential to do this if you want to write a good literature review. The marker will want you to demonstrate that you are developing the ability to construct an argument, which requires you to include only material that is directly relevant to the points that you are making.

How far should I go back?

How far you go back depends entirely upon your research focus; for example, including classic studies could be highly relevant for some research projects. You can include a time limit on how far you go back, but you need to provide a justification for this; sometimes modules will specify a time limit such as within the last ten years. Whichever approach you take, you are expected to have a good grasp of current developments. If you have no material from the last ten years, it may appear that you have not developed your literature-searching skills sufficiently. It is possible that there really is no literature from the last decade, but you need to explain this and what measures you have taken to find it.

What if I search for literature relating to my topic and there is not a great deal out there?

It is always helpful to be explicit in your dissertation about how you conducted your literature search. For example, 'I used the MEDLINE, Cochrane and Applied Social Sciences Index Abstracts (ASSIA) databases using the following search terms: *x, y, z.*'

This makes the process transparent and enables the reader to see exactly what you did. This is particularly important if the literature that you identify is rather limited, because it helps convince the reader that you have undertaken a concerted and systematic attempt to identify relevant material. If your literature is extremely sparse, you need to consider whether you've chosen a suitable topic for your project, because it can be difficult to write your literature review and for you to discuss the significance of your findings without responding to a body of literature, and it can be complex and confusing using related but not directly relevant literature to construct an argument.

What if my original literature review does not cover (or match) all of the issues that came out in the data?

If your literature review forms part of an empirical research study, you may find that you need to revise your literature review because your data have highlighted issues that were not in your original literature review. This is quite common in qualitative studies, where your research is more exploratory. Occasionally there can be a serious mismatch between the original literature review and the issues identified in the data analysis which requires a significant reworking of the literature review. The most common reason for this is that the questions used at data collection stage (e.g. interview or focus group questions) were not clearly linked into the literature review so they cover different topics. Once the data are analysed, the issues raised need to be the focus of a revised literature review. The simplest remedy is to ensure that your data collection questions are informed by and relate to the issues identified in your literature review. For most research projects, the revisions are relatively minor but do ensure that you allow yourself sufficient time at the writing-up stage.

Chapter summary

In this chapter, we looked at how to write up a literature review. We examined the different purposes of a literature review, both as a stand-alone piece of work and as part of an empirical research project. We looked at different ways of structuring your literature review and explored how reference management software can be helpful.

There were a number of key messages. Ensure that you provide a clear account of how you undertook your literature search so that the reader knows that your search was systematic and rigorous. It is important that you signpost your literature review at each stage, so readers know what to expect and what you have already covered.

Activity: Brief outline answer

Activity 10.1   Critical thinking (page 184)

As a first draft, Folashade's original statement is too much like a list of the available literature rather than a critical appraisal of it. Studies are described separately, with no attempt to create an overall narrative. An alternative paragraph could be:

> *Culture can have an important role to play in child protection in several ways. Firstly, the culture of a country can influence whether particular parental behaviour is defined as abusive, e.g. neglect is much less recognised in mainland China than in many European countries (Qiao et al., 2018). Secondly, it can affect particular minority ethnic communities within a wider culture, such as child abuse linked to beliefs in witchcraft and spirit possession within African communities in London (Briggs and Whittaker, 2018). However, Wills et al. (2017) found that culture needed a great emphasis in many government initiatives. Finally, it must be recognised that culture is not only related to race and ethnicity but can include other forms of culture, such as Deaf culture (Evans and Whittaker, 2010).*

If this issue was central to Folashade's research question, she would discuss it in more detail and would probably write a paragraph for each study and discuss methodological issues in depth.

Further reading

Aveyard, H (2023) *Doing a Literature Review in Health and Social Care* (5th edition). Berkshire: Open University Press.

A useful and rigorous account of conducting a literature review.

Hart, C (2018) *Doing a Literature Review: Releasing the Social Science Research Imagination* (2nd edition). London: Sage.

A classic text on compiling your literature review that gives detailed guidance on structure and evaluating arguments.

Useful websites

www.casp-uk.net

The Critical Appraisal Skills Programme (CASP) supports an evidence-based approach in health and social care and has developed a number of tools to help with the process of critically appraising articles. The website contains evaluation tools for a range of approaches, including systematic reviews, randomised controlled trials, qualitative research, economic evaluation studies and diagnostic test studies.

Chapter 11 Writing your research proposal and dissertation

Chapter aims

After reading this chapter, you should be able to:

- feel confident about writing up your dissertation;
- feel confident about writing a proposal;
- understand the different skills needed for presenting quantitative and qualitative research.

Introduction

In this chapter we will do two things: we will introduce you to some basic skills in writing (relating these to writing a dissertation), and we will give you some tips about how to write a research proposal. As most of this book has been written from the perspective of planning a project, including tips on how to write up a finished project may seem odd, but these points are relevant to anyone writing a large and extensive piece of work. Indeed, in some institutions an extended study such as a research proposal and literature review are considered to be a form of dissertation, even though no data have been collected.

We will look first at skills relevant to writing a dissertation, including some general advice about writing per se, before finishing off with looking at specific issues relating to a proposal. The differences between presenting quantitative and qualitative research will be outlined.

Writing a dissertation

A dissertation or research proposal and literature review is likely to be the longest piece of independent work that you will submit for your course, so compliance with the university's requirements is essential. Not all university degree programmes contain a dissertation so be sure to read the guidelines on what your university requires.

The process of writing

Writing up your research dissertation can be both exciting and daunting because it is unlike your previous coursework in three ways. First, it has a structure and terminology that are unlike the standard essay format. Second, it is likely to be a long piece of work, longer than an essay and usually completed with some element of self-directed study over a longer time period than normal. Third, it is likely that you will have some form of one-to-one tutorial support from a lecturer; this is often called supervision.

The writing process itself can be a source of anxiety. Becker describes running a seminar on writing skills and found that students identified two main fears:

> *They were afraid that they would not be able to organise their thoughts, that writing would be a big, confused chaos that would drive them mad. They spoke feelingly about a second fear, that what they wrote would be 'wrong' and that (unspecified) people would laugh at them.*

(Becker, 2007, page 4)

Becker (2007) found that students adopted a number of coping mechanisms to manage their anxiety. For example, using particular pens or paper, sharpening pencils, or cleaning the house (he found a gender divide on the latter).

Activity 11.1 Reflection

Can you relate to these fears? Are there different concerns and anxieties you have about writing?

As this activity is for your own reflection, there is no outline answer given.

You may have been able to see yourself in Becker's comments. Or there may be other anxieties and concerns that you were able to identify. The important point is not to let yourself be paralysed by your anxieties.

One common barrier is the belief that you must read everything that is written on your topic and work out your ideas before you put them down. The danger is that writing will be continually postponed while you read and think some more. Start writing as soon as you can because the writing process helps to identify your thoughts. Becker expresses it well:

> *Writing a dissertation starts with writing, not with preparing to write … And feeling unready is no excuse at all. In scholarship, one is never ready, since there is always something else that one can sensibly read. All scholarship, strictly speaking, is at first written by the unprepared, or at least by the under-prepared. Since you are never ready to write, you start writing before you are ready.*
>
> (Becker, 1986, page 88)

Delamont et al. (2004) offer two golden rules for writing your dissertation:

1. Write early and write often: the more you write, the easier it gets, and it becomes a habit. The later you leave it to start writing, the more difficult it can become. Work out the times that you are most productive and try to develop a routine of writing something every day.

2. Don't get it right, get it written: drafting is an essential stage in working out what you want to say. In previous smaller essays on single topics, it may have been possible to hold everything in your head while you plan. With a dissertation, you have simply too much material, and often a series of related topics that you progressively develop, so drafting is an essential part of the process of working out what you want to say. As you write, you are likely to see some of the tensions, contradictions and inconsistencies in your argument (Delamont et al., 2004, page 121).

Free writing, in which you write down whatever comes into your head without censoring or editing, can help you to establish what you want to say without being paralysed by choices (Becker, 2007). It also helps you realise that you can write your ideas down without fear, and that the only draft that counts is the final draft.

Activity 11.2   Reflection

Write for 5–10 minutes about your thoughts and feelings concerning writing up your dissertation and what barriers you envisage. If you run out of things to say, repeat your last word continuously until further words come to you.

As this activity is for your own reflection, there is no outline answer given.

This is a useful exercise for two reasons. First, you experience the process of free writing and discover how liberating and frightening it can be to write whatever comes into your head. It can be a powerful lesson in how we often do not know what we think about a subject until we see what we have written down on the page. Second, the content of what you have written helps you to understand the potential barriers to you completing your dissertation. These barriers can be physical; for example, finding and protecting the time given the other demands of the course and your personal and work life. They can also be psychological, such as the fear that you will not be able to produce academic work of the standard required. This fear is particularly common and can partly explain why dissertations are often delayed more than other pieces of coursework (although other reasons, such as delays in getting ethical approval or access to participants, are at least as important). Identifying these barriers will help you plan to overcome them.

One common way of planning your writing is to use a SWOT analysis (strengths, weaknesses, opportunities, and threats; this is sometimes called a SCOT analysis, with C standing for challenges, but the principle is the same). If you are engaged in writing a dissertation, literature review and/or proposal, right at the very beginning sit down and spend a couple of hours writing a SWOT analysis. Include some concrete objectives with each element, giving them a time frame as you work towards the final submission date. You might want to think about your skills in relation to the following areas:

- literature searching;
- critiquing research reports;
- concepts of evidence-based practice and clinical effectiveness;
- qualitative research concepts and methods;
- quantitative research concepts and methods;
- writing a research proposal;
- personal study skills and time management;
- use of information technologies.

Structuring your dissertation or proposal

Your university will provide you with specific guidelines for how to structure your dissertation, research proposal or project, and these will be in the relevant module handbook or study guide. Make sure that you adhere to them to the letter. This is particularly true if your university has developed a structure that is specific to that module or programme. However, most universities use a traditional dissertation format and provide less detailed guidance, so this chapter will be important for helping you know how to structure your work.

The traditional dissertation layout has the format given below. A proposal will not have a findings section, but instead may include sections on clinical relevance, dissemination, and risks to the project:

1. Title page: check your university's rules about the exact format.

2. Table of contents: this provides a clear guide to where readers can find particular sections.

3. Abstract: this provides a summary of your research, including a brief account of your research design and findings. In a proposal there will not be any findings.

4. Introduction: this should introduce your research question and explain why it is important. It should outline your approach and clarify the structure of the dissertation.

5. Literature review: this is a coherent and critical account of the literature that provides an overall argument based upon your reading of the literature.

6. Methodology: this explains in clear and specific terms how you conducted your research. It includes an overview of what you did, why you made your choices and how you addressed ethical issues. For proposals these will be in the future tense ('I plan to use an action research methodology').

7. Findings and discussion: in quantitative dissertations, the presentation of findings is usually separated from the discussion section, while they are combined for qualitative research.

8. Conclusion: the conclusion should summarise your research and its major components together with a summary of the principal findings and how they relate to the literature. The conclusion could include recommendations for policy and practice and for future research, listing possible areas of inquiry.

9. References: these should be set out in the appropriate format for your university.

10. Appendices: these include additional background information, such as your interview schedule or questionnaire and sample information sheets given to participants.

Writing your abstract

Although your abstract appears first, it is best to write this last. Abstracts are commonly 250–350 words and the aim is to condense your research project into a short summary. Your abstract contains the basic message of your research and should include your research question or topic, methodology, findings, and their significance for the field.

Look at the journal articles that you have read for your literature review. Each contains an abstract that is carefully crafted because the authors know that most readers will search the literature using bibliographic databases containing abstracts only. If the abstract is badly written and unclear, few readers will take the time to read the whole article. Use them as examples to inform your writing. Some journals (like the *Journal of Advanced Nursing* and the *Journal of Clinical Nursing*) also have a summary section which asks authors to indicate what is already known and what this piece adds. This might be useful as part of the abstract, as might the inclusion of three or four key words.

Writing your introduction

This should introduce your research question and explain why it is important. Stating that it is a long-standing interest for you is not enough on its own, although this could be part of a rationale for undertaking the study. Indeed, frequently students will be asked to choose an area from their practice that they want to investigate further. This gives it a personal, clinical focus that is highly valuable in nursing.

As a general guide, your introduction should start with your main aims and provide a short summary of the background context of your study. Frequently there is a policy context that should be acknowledged in the introduction, whereas the literature review section will review a body of research literature, systematic reviews and guidelines (if there are any). The introduction should be clear about the main problem or issues to be investigated and present your overall approach. Finally, you should provide a short description of the structure of your dissertation (Walliman, 2016).

You do not have to start writing by working on the introduction. Indeed, there are good arguments for writing your introduction last, because it is at that stage that you will have a good idea of what you are going to say. It is not uncommon to read dissertation introductions that state that a particular topic will be discussed, then find that the main body of the dissertation is about a different topic. This is usually because the writer has developed their thinking and discovered that the research is really about the second topic rather than the first topic. This is a healthy part of the research process, but you need to ensure that you redraft your introduction to reflect this.

Writing your literature review

Chapter 10 covers this in detail but, to recap, a popular approach is the chronological structure, which begins with the early development of the field and progresses through to the most recent developments. For example, Christina is a child health nursing student on placement in a hospital ward who is interested in interprofessional working when there are concerns about a child's welfare (see Chapter 3). Her literature review discusses previous writing on interprofesssional working. She could adopt a chronological structure that examines how the topic has been discussed during different time periods.

Alternatively, Christina could adopt a thematic approach that focuses on particular issues identified in the literature, such as challenges in interprofessional communication or differences in organisational policies. This could have a funnel structure, looking at the wider context of policy and practice across different health and social care settings and progressively narrowing down to interprofesssional working when there are concerns about a child's welfare. Either structure is acceptable and good dissertations will give a clear rationale for the structure selected.

Some universities might expect you to conduct a systematic review of the literature. In that case you will need to give search terms, databases and numbers of hits, and your inclusion and exclusion criteria. It may be possible to discuss findings from this approach chronologically, but a thematic structure would be more impressive, so that you can group papers by their underlying theme. These can be summarised in an appendix to indicate how thoroughly you have reviewed the literature, as shown in Table 11.1.

Rather than taking things at face value, a good literature review will address the contradictions and omissions in previous writing. Remember that what scores highly (and will probably be a module requirement in the last year of an undergraduate programme or in postgraduate studies) is a critical analysis and synthesis of the literature. So, what are your papers indicating as a body of literature? Are there key themes or issues to be identified? Are there strengths and weaknesses in their methodologies? What is the impact for your study of the methodological approach taken in the papers? (If you find only small-scale qualitative studies, is it time for a large-scale quantitative design, for example?)

Table 11.1   How to present a brief summary of papers as an appendix

Full reference	Study aims and design	Methods of data collection and analysis	Results	Comments
Lock CA, Kaner E, Heather N, Doughty J, Crawshaw A, McNamee P, Purdy S & Pearson P (2006) Effectiveness of nurse-led brief alcohol intervention: a cluster randomized controlled trial. Journal of Advanced Nursing 54 (4): 426–439.	A pragmatic cluster randomised controlled trial was carried out to evaluate the effects of a brief intervention compared with standard advice (the control group).	Excessive consumption was identified opportunistically via the Alcohol Use Disorders Identification Test. After baseline assessment, patients received either a 5–10-minutes brief intervention using the 'Drink Less' protocol or standard advice (control condition). Follow-up occurred at 6- and 12-months post-intervention.	There were no statistically significant differences between intervention and control patients at follow-up.	
And so on.				

Avoid phrases such as 'research tells us' unless you are prepared to state exactly which research studies you are referring to and provide some form of critical analysis of them. Your marker is unlikely to let vague references to unspecified research go unchallenged at this stage in your studies.

Writing your methodology section

Journalists are taught that the first sentence of a newspaper article should answer the following questions: who, what, when, where, why and sometimes how (Leki, 1998, page 25). While academic readers are likely to be more forgiving, these questions are useful to guide your methodology section. Your methodology section should usually address the following areas:

- Overall research approach and methods: what is/was your overall approach (qualitative or quantitative)? This is often referred to as your choice of paradigm and can also be termed the choice of methodology (as distinct from your methods). What research methods will you/did you use to collect your data (interviews, questionnaires, focus groups)? Why did you choose this approach and research method compared to alternative approaches?
- Sampling: who will/did you have as participants? What is/was the size and composition of your sample? How will/did you select and contact them? Where will/did you go to get access to them?
- Analysis: how will/did you analyse your data? Why will/did you choose that particular approach?
- Ethical issues: how will/did you address ethical issues, such as gaining access to participants or other sources of data, informed consent, confidentiality, anonymising data and ethical data management?
- Limitations: what are the limitations of your research? This discussion can begin here and be developed further in the discussion of your findings.

Presenting and discussing your qualitative data

Obviously if you have not collected data, you won't be doing this, but there are some points here that might inform your thinking about presenting qualitative data. In qualitative dissertations, the presentation of findings is in prose form and lends itself to being discussed immediately. Consequently, findings and discussion are usually combined into one section.

In Chapter 5, thematic analysis was outlined as a good model for analysing most forms of qualitative data. The six-stage model developed by Braun and Clarke (2006) was outlined and the first five stages were described in detail. Our focus in this chapter is on the final stage, writing up and presenting your analysis.

The final stage begins when you have established and refined your themes. Your task in writing up your analysis is to tell the complicated story of your data in a way which convinces the reader of the merit and validity of your analysis (Braun and Clarke, 2006, page 93). Your aim is to provide a concise and coherent narrative that contains sufficient quotes that demonstrate your themes without becoming repetitive. Do not present your quotes without explanation and expect readers to make the connections themselves. Just as you would make an argument and provide a quote from a book or article as evidence to strengthen your argument, use the quotes from your participants in a similar way. Choose particularly vivid and concise quotes that demonstrate your point as closely as possible. Better to have one or perhaps two crisp quotes than include three or four more general quotes. Your quotes need to illustrate a narrative that presents an argument about how the data respond to your research question.

Your findings should be organised according to the themes identified in your analysis rather than just using your interview or focus group questions as a structure. If you just summarise what participants said in response to question one, two and so on, this presents an impression that you have merely described your data rather than analysed them. Avoid using statistics to present your findings when you have small sample sizes. Stating '80 per cent of participants' sounds more dramatic than 'four out of five participants' but your reader is aware of your sample size and is unlikely to be convinced.

The key ethical issue in your findings section is protecting the confidentiality of your participants. The highest risk is often when you use a quote and identify a participant by a characteristic, such as the person's role, gender, ethnicity, or sexual orientation. If the group that the participant belongs to is small, there is a high risk that other participants or other interested parties would be able to identify them. Consequently, avoid identifying a participant in this way; it rarely detracts significantly from your analysis. If you feel that you must, you may need to show your final draft to the participant to obtain their permission.

Presenting and discussing your quantitative data

We have looked at descriptive and inferential statistics in Chapter 7, so what follows are some general points about presenting quantitative data. In quantitative research, the presentation of findings is in table and graph form, so it is conventional to split findings and discussion into two separate headings. A common practice is to include your raw data as an appendix at the back and draw upon the key data in the main body of your dissertation to illustrate your argument. Charts and tables should be in the body of the text, not as an appendix, otherwise it is difficult for readers to follow your argument.

Make your presentation of data attractive and clear. Always give a chart a title and make sure it is clear what it represents. Mark the axes to show scale and include legends to indicate figures or percentages. For a detailed discussion of the presentation of quantitative data, see Dunleavy (2003).

Although the general principles of presenting quantitative data are straightforward, it can take time to get it right. Indeed, Delamont et al. (2003) argue that you should 'expect to suffer' about the presentation of statistics. Although this may be pessimistic, do allow yourself sufficient time. It is likely that you will run various tests over and over again as you develop understanding of the possibilities of your computer program and your thinking develops about the study itself.

In quantitative research, a separate discussion section enables you to examine the significance of your findings. This can be compared to other studies or to theories in your field. The discussion of your findings enables you to revisit your original research question and explore what you have learnt.

Avoid over-generalising your findings. What you may find in one setting in one area at one point in time can rarely be generalised to all populations at all points in time and it is important to be clear about this in your findings section. Silverman captures this eloquently:

> *It always helps to make limited claims about your own research. Grandiose claims about originality, scope or applicability to social problems are all hostages to fortune. Be careful in how you specify the claims of your approach. Show that you understand that it constitutes one way of 'slicing the cake' and that other approaches, using other forms of data, may not be directly competitive.*

(Silverman, 2017, page 49)

In research, it is always wise to be realistic about what you can claim based upon your evidence and better to understate rather than overstate your findings.

For both forms of data analysis, in your discussion make sure that you are clear about how your findings answer your research questions, and make sure that you link and discuss how your study sits in relation to the body of literature. This can be done by noting how your findings equate with other work in the field and may involve you revisiting some of the literature you used to justify the study in the literature review section. It may also require you to draw on extra references to literature that you have not already discussed.

Writing your conclusion

The conclusion should summarise your research and its major components together with a summary of the principal findings and how it relates to the literature. You should not introduce new material at this stage but should summarise complex arguments you have given in the discussion. Your conclusion could discuss lessons learnt from the process of research as well as the findings. Your conclusion could include recommendations for education, policy and practice in your research area. It could also include recommendations for future research, listing possible areas of inquiry or research designs. Try to be specific rather than simply stating that 'further research should be done'.

Some general points

Should I use 'I' in my dissertation?

Traditionally, students were encouraged to use the passive voice; for example, 'the research interviews were conducted with six participants', rather than the active voice, 'I conducted interviews with six participants'. Students were particularly instructed to avoid using 'I' because it appeared too informal and not compatible with the 'scientific' tone expected. Within quantitative research using a positivist approach, this convention is usually still observed, though the active voice is more acceptable than using 'I'. In qualitative research, the active voice is encouraged, and 'I' is used more frequently, because reflexivity is actively encouraged.

Your choice should be guided by whether your research is quantitative or qualitative and by the expectations of your university and supervisor. If you do choose to use 'I', use it sparingly. Avoid overuse; for example, 'I think that I found that I was approaching my topic because I feel I had previously viewed my beliefs ...'. Use 'I' when it genuinely adds something to what you are saying.

Structuring your dissertation

This is not just about headings. A good dissertation includes clear signposting. Since you are taking your reader on a journey, it is important to provide clear statements about where you are going and where you have been. At the end of each section, recap and tell the reader what you will be discussing next.

The function of sentences and paragraphs

A sentence is used to express a single idea. If a sentence expresses two or more ideas, you are probably making it work too hard. Try splitting it into two sentences for greater clarity.

A paragraph consists of several sentences grouped together to express a set of related ideas. Consequently, one-sentence paragraphs are to be avoided.

Knowing what to leave out

Do not feel that you have to use every piece of material that you have gathered through the research process. The marker will want you to show you can construct an argument and use material selectively. This requires you to leave out material that is not relevant, which is much better than trying to 'shoehorn' extraneous material into your dissertation because you have expended considerable effort in obtaining it. A good researcher knows that the quality of research is as much about what is left out as what is included.

Referencing and proofreading your work

Referencing in your dissertation is no different to an essay or another piece of academic work. Most UK universities have adopted the Harvard referencing system and have produced help sheets to provide guidance. Check with your university website or library. Even if you know the Harvard system well, it is worthwhile checking because there are minor differences between universities about how they have interpreted the Harvard system. Many students feel that this is relatively unimportant, but good referencing does impress markers, so it is well worth learning how to reference accurately.

One of the most common mistakes is for your references to omit texts that you have cited and to include texts that you have not cited. This is usually because you have included your references as you have worked on your drafts, but not checked them at the end. So, as you have reworked your material, you have cut out material but left the original references in. Conversely, you have included material that cites texts that you have not yet put in your references. This mismatch between dissertation and references is surprisingly common, even with otherwise diligent students. To check you have the right references in it, it is useful to go through each page, making sure that those that are there are listed in the reference section.

As you write, ensure that you save your work frequently and keep back-up copies. As a general rule, keep a back-up copy on one or more removable drives and e-mail yourself a copy regularly. This ensures that, even if your computer and removable drives were destroyed, you would still have a copy of your work.

Finally, careful proofreading is always worthwhile because it makes it easier for readers to understand what you are saying. Try to complete your dissertation before the deadline. This enables you to sleep on it and reread your dissertation with fresh eyes. Ideally, enlist another person because they are more likely to identify mistakes or confusions that you may miss.

If you have checked your spelling and grammar, markers are more likely to notice what you have to say, rather than being distracted by poor presentation and typing mistakes. Coco Chanel reputedly said: *Dress shabbily and they remember the dress; dress impeccably and they remember the woman.* The same is true of writing.

Disseminating and publishing your work

Completing your dissertation is a significant achievement. Having met the requirements of your degree, it may be tempting just to put it proudly on your bookshelf. However, it is worth considering how to disseminate your research to a wider audience. Managers, colleagues, service users and carers are all stakeholders who could benefit from hearing the results of your research. This can range from a presentation or short summary to writing for a professional or academic publication. If you are considering this, speak to your supervisor, who may be able to provide useful help and advice. It is unlikely that a student could get a piece published in a reputable academic journal without help, so an experienced academic with a good publication record in that type of journal should help you. Your supervisor might suggest that you try to publish if your work is good. In that case, the usual arrangement is that you would take first authorship and the supervisor second. If you enjoyed your research project, you may also want to discuss opportunities for further research with your supervisor, either independently or as a part of further study.

Having looked at writing skills that are relevant to any type of writing, we will now examine some tips specifically for proposal writing.

Proposal writing tips

Wong (2002) has a number of suggestions that relate specifically to proposal writing. He argues that students frequently do not understand how important a proposal is and how its quality influences one's chances of success: without knowing what you are doing in advance and having clearly defined your methodology and methods of data collection and analysis, you will be adrift without a compass when it comes to actually doing the work. A proposal should show that your research is worth doing and that you have the knowledge and skills to complete it successfully: apart from these practicalities, it is unethical for an institution to allow students to undertake research if they don't know how or why they are collecting data, or what they are going to do with it, as this exposes participants to unnecessary, unjustified or unwise procedures. Obviously, then, your proposal should contain all the elements involved in the research process, with enough material at the correct level for your programme of study so that readers and markers can assess why the study is needed, what you plan to do and how you plan to do it (Wong, 2002). This can be achieved by a thorough literature review and critical analysis, accurate and appropriate specification of the methodology and methods, addressing ethical considerations rather than just saying 'ethical approval will be obtained', and writing in a structure that addresses the assessment and/or institutional requirements. It should also be written in a coherent and engaging manner that has correct standards of English, grammar and punctuation, and has been effectively proofread. Another useful tip is to get someone with more experience to read it. This could be a researcher or, more likely for students, a supervisor or module lecturer. The title is also very important and should be informative, convey clearly what the proposal is about, reflect the overall methodological approach, and usually (although not necessarily) be a sentence with a question mark at the end. As always, the question drives the study design, not the other way around.

Box 11.1:   How different titles can convey entirely different methodological approaches in proposals

1.   What are the differences in effectiveness between ACE inhibitors and angiotension II receptor blockers?

Comment 1

This question is clearly asking whether there are differences between groups. The researchers want to know which type of intervention works best, so they would construct a null hypothesis that there are no differences between groups and seek to falsify (disprove) it. Methodologically, the way to assess this is to use an experimental design; thus the question drives the choice of study design, not the other way around.

2.   What are patients' experiences of living with long-term hypertension?

Comment 2

Here, there is no sense in which a hypothesis can be tested, as the question is asking for patients' experiences. A qualitative study design would be used in order to get a rich and in-depth perspective of what it is like to live with hypertension in the long term. Individual interviews could be used, with data transcribed and thematically analysed.

3.   How satisfied are patients with hypertension inventions in primary care?

Comment 3

This is a different issue from the two above as the researchers are trying to evaluate a service from the perspective of patients. This could be done using a questionnaire survey. It is neither an experimental design or an in-depth qualitative approach, but could use an existing satisfaction measure, or a specially designed one, using a mix of Likert-scale questions with some free-text open-ended ones.

4.   How effective are nurse-led hypertension clinics? An observational study.

Comment 4

This question contains specific reference to the method to be used, which is observation. This makes it completely clear what the researchers are planning to do and leaves the reader in no doubt about what to expect from the proposal.

Timetable

Every proposal must include a timetable. This shows the time frame to which you will be working. This is most important in any setting, but particularly so if you have to meet coursework deadlines. You will need to plan carefully, and plan on a weekly or monthly basis each step that you will take. Most proposals will have clear steps that mirror the research process, and you will need to allocate these times for starting and finishing. Figure 3.2 on page 54 shows how you can construct a simple timetable using a Microsoft Word table. A more sophisticated and impressive way of presenting your timetable is to use a Gantt chart. Figure 11.1 shows an example of a Gantt chart.

There are many different software packages freely available for doing this if you search the internet, and it can also be achieved using Microsoft Excel.

Resources

A proposal will also need some estimation of resources. If you were submitting your proposal for funding, this would need to be very accurate. Universities and NHS Trusts have teams of dedicated staff to do this, and you should ask them to do it for you if you are looking for funding in reality. Universities are now subject to something called Full Economic Costing (FEC) in research bids and this is a complicated area, so let the accountants get it right for you. In a student's proposal, it would be necessary only to estimate, not cost, the types of resources you might need, such as staff, computers, statistician time, room rental, travel and subsistence costs, and so on.

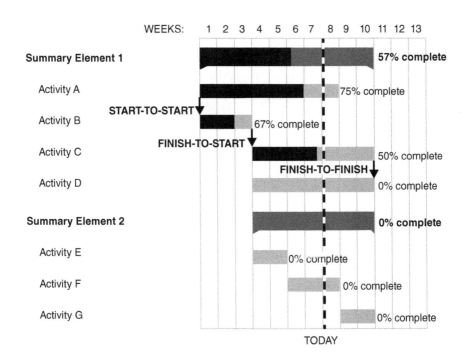

Figure 11.1 Gantt chart for project planning. Adapted from an original diagram by Garry L. Booker (8 October 2007)

Benefits and risks

Some proposal structures will ask you to discuss the benefits of your research, and this can be listed for the local NHS services, nationally and possibly even internationally (although you may need to wait until you are a professor before your work has impact internationally). You may also be asked to list risks in terms of the research to patients, but also in terms of the research not being completed: what happens if you can't recruit? Do you have a plan B?

Dissemination

Finally, it is time for you to think about the best way to publicise your work. Can it be published as a report, or as an article or chapter in a larger academic publication? Could you present your findings at a conference or write it up for a project website? The opportunities are wide-ranging.

Chapter summary

In this chapter, the key messages are to start writing early and to use the writing process to help you work out what you want to say. Do not expect to be able to submit your first draft. You will usually need to draft material more than once before it is ready. SWOT analysis can be used to identify and overcome problems, will give you confidence in areas that you are good at and may be useful in setting personal milestones.

Adopt the structure given by your university and explain it in your introduction. Check with your supervisor and university in the early stages whether your interpretation of the structure is acceptable. In addition to your headings, you should guide the reader through it with clear 'signposting' (i.e. explaining at each stage the stage that has been reached and what you are going to discuss next). Finally, try to get your dissertation ready before the deadline to allow time for a final proofread as this will pay dividends.

Remember that a good research proposal shows examiners that you are competent to carry out the research effectively and ethically. Use your overall question to signpost examiners about your methodological stance and use your literature to argue and justify your study and your methods.

Further reading

Becker, H (2007) *Writing for Social Scientists: How to Start and Finish Your Thesis, Book or Article* (2nd edition). Chicago, IL: University of Chicago Press.

A classic text that provides a very readable and entertaining account of the writing process.

Locke, LF, Spirduso, WW and Silverman, SJ (2014) *Proposals That Work: A Guide for Planning Dissertations and Grant Proposals* (6th edition). Thousand Oaks, CA: Sage.

Gives information on funding grant applications.

Offredy, M and Vickers, P (2010) *Developing a Healthcare Research Proposal: An Interactive Student Guide*. Oxford: Wiley-Blackwell.

Student-focused text.

Punch, K (2016) *Developing Effective Research Proposals* (3rd edition). London: Sage.

Good book with more detail on writing proposals.

Thomas, D and Hodges, ID (2010) *Designing and Planning Your Research Project*. London: Sage.

More detail on writing proposals.

Walliman, NSR (2013) *Your Undergraduate Dissertation: The Essential Guide for Success* (2nd edition). London: Sage.

More tips on effective writing.

Useful websites

www.birmingham.ac.uk/schools/law/courses/research/research-proposal.aspx

Birmingham University Study Guide on how to write a research proposal.

https://www.ncbi.nlm.nih.gov/pmc/articles/PMC5037942/

Hawaii University module (Econ 730) site: useful, with lots of links on proposal writing.

Conclusion

In this book we have presented a wide variety of material that will help you to undertake research literature searching and reviewing, research proposal writing and planning systematic reviews. The emphasis has been on helping you to gain underpinning knowledge, which you can then use for your final-year assignments or dissertations concerning project planning and literature reviewing. Planning research may seem an unlikely task for a student nurse, hoping soon to be a newly qualified staff nurse, but it should be remembered that the 'point' of these assignments is as much about developing transferable skills as it is about formulating research proposals.

In your new role, you will quickly be expected to take on clinical leadership roles, particularly if, as seems likely, you will quickly be expected to supervise Band 4 staff and other unregistered staff as one of only a few Band 5 nurses and above in a shift. Clinical leadership is about skills, attributes and personality, but it is first and foremost about excellent clinical practice, and in order to be able to identify excellent clinical practice, rather than simply operating on 'custom and practice', or 'we always do it like that', you need to have the knowledge to find and appraise evidence, including primary research reports and systematic reviews. The report of the Willis Commission states:

> Graduate nurses, as future leaders of clinical teams, should understand how to evaluate, utilise and conduct research, and act on evidence to improve the quality of care.

(Willis Commission, 2012, page 36)

These are skills that have been outlined in this book. They are important generic skills that you can apply to any aspect of clinical practice of your interest. As you become more senior it is likely that you will take on greater responsibilities than nurses have had previously, with greater autonomy, and even possibly independent prescribing rights: treatment decisions will be yours alone, and in order to make the correct choices for your patients you will need to be able to understand the studies that indicate different options. Also, patients are very well informed these days via the internet, and you will need to be able to evaluate the quality of information they present to you about their illnesses and treatments in order to be clinically credible to them. Will you be able to tell them why an article in a popular magazine, or an internet advert, is of less value in making treatment decisions than a Cochrane systematic review or NICE guidelines? After reading this book you should be able to.

The second element of this book is about planning research projects. Again, you may argue that you'll never be doing research yourself, but you will find as your career progresses that you are expected to undertake further qualifications as part of your work role, or in order to gain promotion. It is apparent from our experience in education that many candidates for Master's degrees have very little background in understanding and applying research methods effectively, and this puts them at a disadvantage compared to other professions that do have that background. We emphasise that it is not learning about research methods that is in itself important, but it is their application in the clinical setting, and this is why you are being asked to plan a project: to show that you understand the existing literature, potential study designs, methods of inquiry and ethical issues sufficiently well. It is also not beyond the realms of possibility that you might be involved with research studies taking place in your workplace, or want to investigate some aspect of clinical care and how to improve it in the future. Nursing will not build a research culture unless clinical nurses identify and investigate clinical questions, and you could be part of that future.

In the Introduction we outlined how this book meets the NMC *Future Nurse: Standards of Proficiency for Registered Nurses* (NMC, 2018), including Annexes A and B, and the Quality Assurance Agency (QAA, 2001) subject benchmarks for nursing. We have not reproduced these in detail again as they are documented in the Introduction. To show how the knowledge and skills you have acquired in this book meet outcomes specifically related to the newly qualified nurse, we would say that we have discussed a range of research methodologies and how to critique literature that uses them; we have discussed how to approach systematic reviews with quantitative and qualitative meta-analyses; and we have outlined how you might construct a proposal using them. Literature searching and project planning can help you to further your knowledge about clinical nursing and evidence-based best practice that relates to the excellent patient care that you aspire to deliver.

One key aspect that all student nurses are interested in is their employability. To that end we have mapped in Table 12.1 the key outcomes from the NHS Knowledge and Skills Framework (Department of Health, 2004) with suggested learning outcomes for undertaking a literature review and proposal module for nurses run by one of us (GW). This indicates that the skills you have learnt by reading this book and undertaking your own modules are rated highly by the NHS for your work role as a newly qualified nurse and are transferable from higher education into the NHS.

Table 12.1 Literature searching and project planning outcomes mapped to the NHS Knowledge and Skills Framework

Module learning outcomes	NHS Knowledge and Skills Framework dimension and level
Undertake a structured, systematic literature search relevant to the chosen topic using electronic databases.	Communication 4c and e. Service development 4b. Quality 3c. Production and communication of information and knowledge 4c, e, f, g, h, i, j. Leadership 3a.
Write a coherent research proposal, exploring methodological issues in study design. Write a critical, integrated literature review on the chosen topic.	Service development 4b and c. Leadership 3a. Research and development 3a, b, c, d, e, f, g, h, i, j. Communication 3b, c, d. Personal and people development 3a, b, c, d, e. Quality 4b. Data processing and management 2e. Production and communication of information and knowledge 3a, c, d, g, i, j; 4e, f, h. Leadership 2a. Research and development 3a, b, c, e, f, g, h, i, j.

Above all, we hope you have enjoyed the book, passed your assignments, projects or dissertations, and are about to qualify for a demanding yet rewarding career as a nurse in your chosen field. The expectations of registrants have never been higher, and we believe passionately that the best nursing practice demands a focus on evidence and research if it is to become more than an aspiration. Good luck.

Glossary

accidental sampling   A lesser-used term for convenience sampling.

action research   An approach that challenges the traditional conception of the researcher as separate from the real world. It is associated with smaller-scale research projects that seek to address real-world problems, particularly among practitioners who want to improve practice. Rather than a specific research method, it is more an approach to research that stresses the importance of links with real-world problems and a belief that research should serve practical ends.

Boolean operators   Specific codes used during electronic literature searches to manipulate your search terms to achieve the best results.

case study   A detailed investigation of a single or small numbers of cases, e.g. an organisation, individual or event. Rather than a research method, it is more a focus of study in which a variety of research methods can be used.

convenience sampling   A form of sampling in which you select your participants on the basis of what is immediately available. This is the least well regarded of sampling strategies.

data   The information that you are going to collect in order to answer your research question. In qualitative research, it is the words used by your participants or contained in texts, whereas in quantitative research data are in numerical form.

empirical data collection or empirical research refers to research involving the collection and analysis of new data.

epistemology   is the study of knowledge and addresses the question of what counts as legitimate knowledge. Every approach to research has underlying assumptions about the nature of knowledge and the social world, which is referred to as an epistemological position. Common approaches are positivism (quantitative research) and interpretivism (qualitative research).

focus group   A group of individuals selected to provide their opinions on a defined subject, facilitated by a moderator who aims to create an open and relaxed environment and promote interaction between participants.

grounded theory   An approach to research that emphasises the importance of generating new concepts and theoretical frameworks from data. Data collection and analysis happen alongside one another and data is analysed as it is collected in a continuous process. This continues until new data do not provide any new insights, the point known as theoretical saturation.

hypothesis   Refers to a theoretical statement about the relationship between two or more variables that predicts an expected outcome. It may be derived from your reading of the literature, a theory or your own observations and experience and must be able to be tested.

interpretivism   A broad term to describe a range of epistemological approaches that challenge the traditional scientific approach of positivism. Interpretivism argues that the research methods of the natural sciences are inappropriate to study social phenomena because they do not take into account the viewpoints of the social actors involved.

interview schedule   A list of questions that you intend to ask in an interview. The equivalent for focus groups is called a discussion guide.

literature review   A comprehensive summary and critical appraisal of the literature that is relevant to your research topic. It presents the reader with what is already known in this field and identifies traditional and current controversies as well as weaknesses and gaps in the field.

literature search   Refers to the initial process of identifying texts that are appropriate using electronic or manual searches. Sometimes treated as if it were synonymous with a literature review.

methodology   Refers to the totality of how you are going to undertake your research. It consists of the research approach that you will use including your epistemological position and the specific research methods you will choose, such as interviews or questionnaires.

multi-stage cluster sampling   A sampling strategy that can be used when a sample is geographically spread. Cluster sampling enables you to group together potential participants and randomly select different sites.

operationalisation   The process of how to convert an abstract concept into a quantifiable measure through deciding which indicators to use when measuring a particular variable.

participants   Replaces the outmoded term 'research subjects' because the latter term suggests that people involved in research should have a passive role in a process to which they are 'subjected'. The term 'participants' suggests a more active and equal role, in which participation is informed and freely chosen.

participatory action research (PAR)   A form of action research that is committed to the involvement of those who are most affected by the issues being studied. It challenges the traditional power imbalance between the researcher as 'expert' and research participant as 'passive subject'.

population   Refers to the total group of people or other units, e.g. documents, which are being researched.

positivism   A view of knowledge in which the methods of the traditional natural sciences are seen as appropriate to the study of social reality. It stresses objectivity and seeks to establish causal relationships. Founded by the sociologist Auguste Comte, it has been influential in quantitative social research.

primary research   Primary research refers to research that involves empirical data collection (e.g. through surveys, interviews or focus groups), while secondary research involves using existing data that has already been collected.

probability or random sampling   Uses mathematical techniques based upon probability theory to select research participants who are representative of the overall population. It is the most commonly used sampling approach used in questionnaire research as randomisation increases the likelihood that the results will be generalisable to a wider population. It has many forms, including simple random sampling, simple stratified sampling and multi-stage cluster sampling.

publication bias   This occurs when the outcome of a study influences whether it will be published. For example, studies that show that an intervention is ineffective may be less likely to be published.

purposive sampling   (sometimes known as judgemental sampling) A popular approach used in qualitative research where participants are chosen because they possess relevant characteristics for the research questions, such as particular experience or knowledge. The aim is to produce theoretical and interesting data rather than statistically generalisable findings.

qualitative research   Tends to emphasise words as data, such as the words of participants in an interview or written data from documents. Rather than seeking to develop specific testable hypotheses, qualitative research seeks to explain the meaning of social phenomena through exploring the ways in which individuals understand their social worlds.

quantitative research   Tends to emphasise quantification and measurement, which can be analysed using statistical tests to establish causal relationships between variables. Has been influenced by positivism as a traditional scientific model, which emphasises 'objectivity' by seeking to remove the values and attitudes of the researcher from the study. Sampling issues are particularly important because of the emphasis on being able to create statistical generalisations that are applicable to the wider population.

quota sampling   Is a procedure in which the researcher decides to research groups or quotas of people from specific subsections of the total population. Common categories are demographic, such as age, gender and ethnicity, but they could be related to the research topic.

randomised controlled trial (RCT)   A classical experimental design, in which participants are randomly assigned to one of two groups: an experimental group and a control group. The experimental group receives the intervention while the control group does not, and the effects are then measured in each group.

reliability   A measure of how consistent or stable a particular measure is.

research approach or paradigm   refers to your overall view of research. A key distinction is between quantitative and qualitative research approaches. Quantitative research uses information in numerical form and has traditionally been influenced by a scientific worldview, most usually positivism. It stresses objectivity and seeks causal explanations. Qualitative research tends to use data in the form of words and seeks to explain the meaning of social phenomena through understanding the ways in which individuals make sense of their social worlds.

research method   Refers to the practical ways that you are going to collect your data. The most commonly used methods in student research are interviews, surveys/questionnaires and focus groups. Each method has a separate chapter.

sampling Refers to the process of selecting the participants (or other data sources, e.g. documents) that will be involved in your study. Your sample (the selection of people or other data sources) is chosen from the total possible data sources, known as the population. Sample refers to the segment of the population that is selected for the research study. Sampling frame refers to a list of all members of the population being researched, e.g. a list of all students at a university or every nurse on the NMC register.

secondary research While primary research refers to research that involves empirical data collection (e.g. through surveys, interviews or focus groups), secondary research involves using existing data that has already been collected.

simple random sampling The most basic form of random sampling in which cases are selected randomly. Each unit of the population has an equal chance of being included in the sample and this method eliminates human bias.

simple stratified sampling Recognises the different strata in a population and aims to select a representative sample by ensuring each section is appropriately represented.

snowball sampling A technique where the researcher selects a small number of participants and asks them to recommend other suitable people who may be willing to participate in the study. This is appropriate when participants are difficult to identify and contact, such as sex workers or people who are homeless.

surveys Used to study large groups or populations, usually using a standardised, quantitative approach to identify beliefs, attitudes, behaviour and other characteristics. Questionnaires form a key research method for collecting survey data, but surveys can use a range of methods, such as highly structured face-to-face or telephone interviews.

systematic review A form of literature review that uses an explicit and transparent set of formal protocols that seek to minimise the chances of systematic bias and error. Historically, these have usually been commissioned by governmental or national bodies in order to provide guidance about specific areas of practice but they are increasingly used in university courses. This usually applies to quantitative work, although there are qualitative, narrative approaches.

systematic sampling A variation of the simple random sample in which cases are selected in a systematic way, e.g. choosing every tenth case.

thematic analysis A popular method for analysing qualitative data by identifying patterns of meaning. It is a versatile and flexible approach that can be used with a range of different qualitative approaches.

theoretical sampling A type of non-probability sampling in which the sample is chosen because it is anticipated to illustrate and lead to further refinement of a theoretical issue. Developed as part of grounded theory, it has been argued that it is effectively synonymous with purposive sampling. Rather than predetermine the number of participants, researchers will carry on interviewing participants until 'saturation' has been achieved, where no significantly new data is being produced and the themes have been exhausted.

validity Refers to whether what we are measuring is what we think we are measuring.

variables Attributes that can take on different values with different cases and could include your participants' attitudes, beliefs, behaviour, knowledge or some other characteristic.

References

Alston, M and Bowles, W (2012) *Research for Social Workers* (3rd edition). St Leonard, NSW: Allen & Unwin.

Andrews, M, Day Sclater, S, Rustin, M, Squire, C and Treacher, A (eds) (2004) *Uses of Narrative*. New Brunswick, NJ: Transition.

Andrews, M, Squire, C and Tamboukou, M (eds) (2013) *Doing Narrative Research* (2nd edition). London: Sage

Atkinson, P and Mukaetova-Ladinska, EB (2012). Nurse-led liaison mental health service for older adults: Service development using lean thinking methodology. *Journal of Psychosomatic Research*, 72(4), 328–31.

Aveyard, H (2023) *Doing a Literature Review in Health and Social Care* (5th edition). Berkshire: Open University Press.

Barthes, R (1972) *Mythologies*. New York: Hill & Wang.

Becker, H (1986) *Writing for Social Scientists: How to Start and Finish Your Thesis, Book or Article*. Chicago, IL: University of Chicago Press.

Becker, H (2007) *Writing for Social Scientists: How to Start and Finish Your Thesis, Book or Article* (2nd edition). Chicago, IL: University of Chicago Press.

Bhaskar, R (1978) *A Realist Theory of Science* (2nd edition). Atlantic Highlands, NJ: Humanities Press.

Bhaskar, R (1979) *The Possibility of Naturalism: A Philosophical Critique of the Contemporary Human Sciences*. Brighton: Harvester.

Bhaskar, R (1990) *Harré and His Critics*. Oxford: Blackwell.

BMJ (2018) Chapter 8. Case-control and cross sectional studies in *Epidemiology for the uninitiated*. Available online at www.bmj.com/about-bmj/resources-readers/publications/epidemiology-uninitiated/8-case-control-and-cross-sectional.

Bowen, S, Erickson, T, Martens, PJ and Crockett, S (2009) More than 'using research': the real challenges in promoting evidence-informed decision-making. *Healthcare Policy*, 4 (3): 87–102.

Boyatzis, RE (1998) *Transforming Qualitative Information: Thematic Analysis and Code Development*. Thousand Oaks, CA: Sage.

Braun, V and Clarke, V (2006) Using thematic analysis in psychology. *Qualitative Research in Psychology*, 3: 77–101.

Braun, V and Clarke, V (2013) *Successful Qualitative Research: A Practical Guide for Beginners*. London: Sage.

Briggs, S and Whittaker, A (2018) Protecting children from faith-based abuse through accusations of witchcraft and spirit possession: understanding contexts and informing practice. *British Journal of Social Work, 48* (8): 2157–75.

Brink, P (2012) Issues of reliability and validity, in J Morse (ed.) *Qualitative Nursing Research: A Contemporary Dialogue.* Revised edition. London: Sage.

Caelli, K, Ray, L and Mill, J (2003) 'Clear as mud': toward greater clarity in generic qualitative research. *International Journal of Qualitative Methods, 2* (2). Article 1. Available online at www.ualberta.ca/~iiqm/backissues/2_2/pdf/caellietal.pdf

Cartwright, N (2007) Are RTCs the gold standard? *Biosocieties, 2*: 11–20.

Chiang, C-Y and Sun, F-K (2009) The effects of a walking program on older Chinese American immigrants with hypertension: a pretest and posttest quasi-experimental design. *Public Health Nursing, 26* (3): 240–8.

Clark, T, Foster, L, Bryman, A and Sloan, L (2021) *Bryman's Social Research Methods* (6th edition). Oxford: Oxford University Press.

Clarke, M (2006) Part 1: Systematic review and meta analysis of quantitative research, overview of methods. Chapter 1 in C Webb and B Roe (eds) *Reviewing Research Evidence for Nursing Practice: Systematic Reviews.* Oxford: Blackwell Publishing, pages 1–8.

Clements, S and Foster, N (2008) Newspaper reporting on schizophrenia: a content analysis of five national newspapers at two time points. *Schizophrenia Research, 98*: 178–83.

Coghlan, D and Brannick, T (2019) *Doing Action Research in Your Own Organisation* (5th edition). London: Sage.

Cook, G (2023) Into a place where thoughts can bloom: A reflection on how raising awareness of our multiple intelligences can support learning and growth. *International Practice Development Journal, 13*(1) doi:https://doi.org/10.19043/ipdj.131.012

Cooke, A, Smith, D and Booth, A (2012) Beyond PICO: the SPIDER tool for qualitative evidence synthesis. *Qualitative Health Research, 22*: 1435–43.

Courtenay, M, Carey, N and Stenner, K (2009) Nurse prescriber–patient consultations: a case study in dermatology. *Journal of Advanced Nursing, 65* (6): 1207–17.

Crandon, S (2017) Case-control and cohort studies: a brief overview. Available online at www.students4bestevidence.net/case-control-and-cohort-studies-overview.

Cresswell, J (2021) *A Concise Introduction to Mixed Methods Research* (2nd edition). London: Sage Publications.

Crossley, M (2000) *Introducing Narrative Psychology: Self, Trauma and Construction of Meaning.* Buckingham: Open University Press.

Crossley, M (2007) Narrative analysis, in E Lyons and A Coyle (eds) *Qualitative Data Analysis in Psychology.* London: Sage.

Curtis, A, Whittaker, A, Stevens, S and Lennon, A (2002) Single session family intervention in a local authority family centre setting. *Journal of Social Work Practice, 16* (1): 37–41.

Daly, J, Willis, K, Small, R, Green, J, Welch, N, Kealy, M and Hughes, E (2007) A hierarchy of evidence for assessing qualitative health research. *Journal of Clinical Epidemiology, 60* (1): 43–49.

Data Protection Act (1998) Available online at www.opsi.gov.uk/Acts/Acts1998/ukpga_19980029_en_1 (13 Feb 2024).

David, M (2006) Editor's introduction, in *Case Study Research: Sage Benchmarks in Social Research Methods*, vol. *1*. London: Sage.

Davies, MB (2007) *Doing a Successful Research Project: Using Qualitative or Quantitative Methods*. Basingstoke: Palgrave Macmillan.

Delamont, S, Atkinson, P and Parry, O (2004) *Supervising the PhD: A Guide to Success* (2nd edition). Buckingham: Open University Press.

Denscombe, M (2014) *The Good Research Guide for Small-Scale Social Research Projects* (5th edition). Buckingham: Open University Press.

Department of Health (2001) *National Service Framework for Older People*. London: HMSO.

Department of Health (2004) *NHS Knowledge and Skills Framework*. Available online at https://webarchive.nationalarchives.gov.uk/ukgwa/20061024094511/http:/www.dh.gov.uk/PublicationsAndStatistics/Publications/PublicationsPolicyAndGuidance/PublicationsPolicyAndGuidanceArticle/fs/en?CONTENT_ID=4009176&chk=WD18ht (accessed 21 July 2010).

Department of Health (2005) *Research Governance Framework for Health and Social Care* (2nd edition). Available online at https://webarchive.nationalarchives.gov.uk/ukgwa/20051219205929/http:/www.dh.gov.uk/assetRoot/04/12/24/27/04122427.pdf (accessed 20 March 2014).

Department of Health (2015) *NHS Constitution for England*. Available online at www.gov.uk/government/publications/the-nhs-constitution-for-england/the-nhs-constitution-for-england#principles-that-guide-the-nhs (accessed 19 February 2024).

Dodds, S, Chamberlain, C and Williamson, GR (2006) Modernising chronic obstructive pulmonary disease admissions to improve patient care: local outcomes from implementing the Ideal Design of Emergency Access project. *Accident and Emergency Nursing, 14* (3): 141–7, doi:10.1016/j.aaen.2006.03.006.

Doll, R and Hill, AB (1954) The mortality of doctors in relation to their smoking habits: a preliminary report. *BMJ, 228*: 1451–5.

Donnan, PT (2015) Experimental research, in D Cormack (ed.) *The Research Process in Nursing* (7th edition). Oxford: Blackwell Science.

Dunleavy, P (2003) *Authoring a PhD: How to Plan, Draft, Write and Finish a Doctoral Thesis or Dissertation*. Basingstoke: Palgrave Macmillan.

Ellen, ME, Léon, G, Bouchard, G, Ouimet, M, Grimshaw, JM and Lavis, JN (2014) Barriers, facilitators and views about next steps to implementing supports for evidence-informed decision-making in health systems: a qualitative study. *Implementation Science, 5*; 9: 179, doi:10.1186/s13012-014-0179-8.

Elliott, J (2005) *Using Narrative in Social Research: Qualitative and Quantitative Approaches.* London: Sage.

Ellis, P (2023) *Evidence-Based Practice in Nursing* (5th edition). London: Sage/Learning Matters.

Epstein, I (2009) *Clinical Data Mining.* Oxford: Oxford University Press.

Epstein, I, Zilberfein, F and Synder, S (1997) Using available information in practice-based outcomes research: a case study of psycho-social risk factors and liver transplant outcomes, in EJ Mullen and JL Magnabosco (eds) *Outcome Measurement in the Human Services: Cross-Cutting Issues and Methods.* Washington, DC: NASW Press, pages 224–33.

Evans, M and Whittaker, A (2010) *Sensory Awareness and Social Work.* Exeter: Learning Matters.

Eysenck, HJ (1995) Problems with meta analysis. Chapter 6 in I Chalmers and DG Altman (eds) *Systematic Reviews.* London: BMJ Publishing Group.

Fealy, GM, McNamara, MS, Casey, M, O'Connor, T, Patton, D, Doyle, L and Quinlan, C (2015) Service impact of a national clinical leadership development programme: findings from a qualitative study. *Journal of Nursing Management, 23* (3): 324–32.

Fitzgerald, L, Ferlie, E, McGivern, G and Buchanan, D (2013) Distributed leadership patterns and service improvement: evidence and argument from English healthcare. *The Leadership Quarterly, 24* (1): 227–39, doi:10.1016/j.leaqua.2012.10.012.

Forster, L, Diamond, I and Banton, J (2014) *Beginning Statistics: An Introduction for Social Scientists* (2nd edition). London: Sage.

Fraser, A, Macdonald-Wallis, C, Tilling, C, Boyd, A, Golding, J, Davey Smith, G, Henderson, J, Macleod, J, Molloy, L, Ness, A, Ring, S, Nelson, SM and Lawlor, DA (2013) Cohort profile: the Avon Longitudinal Study of Parents and Children: ALSPAC mothers cohort. *International Journal of Epidemiology, 42* (1): 97–110, doi.org/10.1093/ije/dys066.

Gibbs, GR (2018) *Analysing Qualitative Data* (2nd edition). London: Sage.

Giddens, A and Sutton, P (2021) *Sociology* (9th edition). Cambridge: Polity Press.

Glaser, B and Strauss, A (1967) *The Discovery of Grounded Theory.* Chicago, IL: Aldine.

Gough, D, Oliver, S and Thomas, J (2017) *An Introduction to Systematic Reviews* (2nd edition). London: Sage.

Graham, ID, Logan, J, Harrison, MB, Straus, SE, Tetroe, J, Caswell, W and Robinson, N (2006) Lost in knowledge translation: time for a map? *The Journal of Continuing Education in the Health Professions, 26* (1): 13–24, doi:10.1002/chp.47.

Gray, DE (2017) *Doing Research in the Real World* (4th edition). London: Sage.

Green, J and Hart, L (1999) The impact of context on data, in Barbour, RS and Kitzinger, J (eds) *Developing Focus Group Research: Politics, Theory and Practice.* London: Sage.

Greenhalgh, T (2014) Evidence based medicine: a movement in crisis? *BMJ, 348*: 3725.

Grimshaw, JM, Eccles, MP, Lavis, JN, Hill, SJ and Squires, JE (2012) Knowledge translation of research findings. *Implementation Science,* 7: 50, doi:10.1186/1748-5908-7-50.

Grol, R and Grimshaw, J (2003) From best evidence to best practice: effective implementation of change in patients' care. *The Lancet, 362,* 9391: 1225–30.

Gubrium, JF and Holstein, JA (2009) *Analysing Narrative Reality.* Thousand Oaks, CA: Sage.

Guyatt, GH (1991) Evidence-based medicine. *ACP Journal Club Archives,* Mar–Apr; *114:* A16, doi:10.7326/ACPJC-1991-114-2-A16.

Happel, B (2007) Focus groups in nursing research: an appropriate method or the latest fad? *Nurse Researcher, 14* (2): 18–24.

Hardiman, M, Connolly, M, Hanley, S, Kirrane, J and O'Neill, W (2020) Designing and implementing an electronic nursing record to support compassionate and person-centred nursing practice in an acute hospital using practice development processes. *Journal of Research in Nursing. 25*(3): 241–53. doi:10.1177/1744987120917719.

Hardiman, M and Dewing, J (2019) Using two models of workplace facilitation to create conditions for development of a person-centred culture: A participatory action research study. *J Clin Nurs. 28*: 2769–81. https://doi.org/10.1111/jocn.14897.

Harrison, MB, Légaré, F, Graham, ID and Fervers, B (2010) Adapting clinical practice guidelines to local context and assessing barriers to their use. *Canadian Medical Association Journal, 182* (2), doi: 10.1503/cmaj.081232.

Hart, C (2018) *Doing a Literature Search: A Comprehensive Guide for the Social Sciences* (2nd edition). London: Sage.

Hemingway, P and Brereton, N (2009) *What is a systematic review?* Bandolier evidence-based medicine series. Available online at https://web.archive.org/web/20231201234511/http://www.bandolier.org.uk/painres/download/whatis/Syst-review.pdf (15 Feb 2024).

Hollis, S and Campbell, F (1999) What is meant by intention to treat analysis? Survey of published randomised controlled trials. *British Medical Journal, 319* (7211): 670–4.

Howick, J (2009) Oxford Centre for Evidence-Based Medicine Levels of Evidence. Produced by Phillips, B, Ball, C, Sackett, D, Badenoch, D, Straus, S, Haynes, B and Dawes, M since November 1998. Updated by Howick, J, March 2009. Available online at www.cebm.ox.ac.uk/resources/levels-of-evidence/oxford-centre-for-evidence-based-medicine-levels-of-evidence-march-2009 (15 Feb 2024).

Huberman, M and Miles, M (2008) Data management and analysis methods, in Denzin, N and Lincoln, Y (eds) *Collecting and Interpreting Qualitative Materials* (3rd edition). London: Sage.

Janis, IL (1982) *Groupthink* (2nd edition). Boston, MA: Houghton Mifflin.

Jordan, Z, Lockwood, C, Aromataris, E and Munn, Z (2016) *The Updated JBI Model for Evidence-Based Healthcare.* The Joanna Briggs Institute.

Khan, SK, Kunz, R, Kleijnan, J and Antes, G (2011) *Systematic Reviews to Support Evidence Based Medicine* (2nd edition). London: Royal Society of Medicine.

Kitson, A, Harvey, G and McCormack, B (1998) Enabling the implementation of evidence-based practice: a conceptual framework. *Quality in Health Care, 7*: 149–58, doi:10.1136/qshc.7.3.149.

Kitson, A, Silverston, H, Wiechula, R, Zeitz, K, Marcoionni, D and Page, T (2011) Clinical nursing leaders', team members' and service managers' experiences of implementing evidence at a local level. *Journal of Nursing Management, 19* (4): 542–55, doi:10.1111/j.1365-2834.2011.01258.x.

Kitson, AL, Rycroft-Malone, J, Harvey, G, McCormack, B, Seers, K and Titchen, A (2008) Evaluating the successful implementation of evidence into practice using the PARiHS framework: theoretical and practical challenges. *Implementation Science, 3*: 1, doi:10.1186/1748-5908-3-1.

Koch, T, Kralik, D, Eastwood, S and Schofield, A (2008) Breaking the silence: women living with multiple sclerosis and urinary incontinence. *International Journal of Nursing Practice, 7* (1): 16–23.

Kralik, D, Price, K, Warren, J and Koch, T (2006) Issues in data generation using email group conversations for nursing research. *Journal of Advanced Nursing, 53* (2): 213–20.

Krueger, RA and Casey, MA (2015) *Focus Groups: A Practical Guide for Applied Research* (5th edition). Thousand Oaks, CA: Sage.

Kübler-Ross, E (1993) *On Death and Dying, first reprint edition.* New York: Collier Books.

Kvale, S (1996) *Interviews: An Introduction to Qualitative Research Interviewing.* London: Sage.

Labov, W and Waletsky, J (1967) Narrative analysis: oral versions of personal experience, in J Helms (ed.) *Essays in the Verbal and Visual Arts.* Seattle, WA: University of Washington.

Lavery, G (2017) Quality improvement - rival or ally of practice development? *International Practice Development Journal, 7*(1) Retrieved from www.proquest.com/scholarly-journals/quality-improvement-rival-ally-practice/docview/1904277397/se-2.

Layder, D (1993) *New Strategies in Social Research.* Cambridge: Polity Press.

Leki, I (1998) *Academic Writing: Exploring Processes and Strategies.* Cambridge: Cambridge University Press.

Liao, Y, Wu, Q, Kelly, BC, Zhang, F, Tang, YY, et al. (2018) Effectiveness of a text-messaging-based smoking cessation intervention ("Happy Quit") for smoking cessation in China: A randomized controlled trial. *PLOS Medicine, 15* (12), e1002713, doi:10.1371/journal.pmed.1002713.

Lincoln, YS and Guba, EG (1985) *Naturalistic Inquiry.* London: Sage.

Lloyd Jones, M (2006) Part 2: Meta-synthesis and meta-study of qualitative research, overview of methods. Chapter 6 in Webb, C and Roe, B (2006) *Reviewing Research Evidence for Nursing Practice: Systematic Reviews.* Oxford: Blackwell Publishing, pages 63–72.

Ludema, JD, Cooperrider, DL and Barrett, FJ (2013) Appreciative inquiry: the power of the unconditional positive question, in Reason, P and Bradbury, H (eds) *Handbook of Action Research* (2nd edition). London: Sage.

Macdonald, J (2003) *Using Systematic Reviews to Improve Social Care,* SCIE Report No. 4. London: Social Care Institute for Excellence.

Mair, M (1989) *Between Psychology and Psychotherapy.* London: Routledge.

Manley, K and McCormack, B (2003) Practice development: purpose, methodology, facilitation and evaluation. *Nursing in Critical Care, 8*: 22–29. https://doi.org/10.1046/j.1478-5153.2003.00003.x.

Marx, K and Griffiths, H (2018) *The Communist Manifesto & Selected Writings'*. Macmillan Collector's Library.

Maxwell, JA (2013) *Qualitative Research Design: An Interactive Approach* (3rd edition). Thousand Oaks, CA: Sage.

McCance, T and McCormack, B (2021) The person-centred practice framework (Chapter 3) in McCormack, B, McCance, T, Bulley, C, Brown, D, McMillan, A and Martin, S (eds) (2021) *Fundamentals of Person-centred Healthcare Practice.* Oxford, UK: Wiley-Blackwell.

McCormack, B (2012) Fundamentals of person-centred healthcare practice, First edition. Wiley Blackwell.

McCormack, B, Rycroft-Malone, J, DeCorby, K, Hutchinson, AM, Bucknall, T, Kent, B, Schultz, A, Snelgrove-Clarke, E, Stetler, C, Titler, M, Wallin, L and Wilson, V (2013) A realist review of interventions and strategies to promote evidence-informed healthcare: a focus on change agency. *Implementation Science, 138*: 107, doi:10.1186/1748-5908-8-107.

McGlynn, EA, Asch, SA, Adams, J, Keesey, J, Hicks, J, DeCristofaro, A and Kerr, EA (2003) The quality of health care delivered to adults in the United States. *New England Journal of Medicine, 348*: 2635–45.

Melnyk, BM, Fineout-Overholt, E, Feinstein, NF, Li, H, Small, L, Wilcox, L and Kraus, R (2004) Nurses' perceived knowledge, beliefs, skills and needs regarding evidence-based practice: implications for accelerating the paradigm shift. *Worldviews on Evidence-Based Nursing, 1* (3): 185–93.

Michell, L (1999) Combining focus groups and interviews: telling how it is, telling how it feels, in Barbour, RS and Kitzinger, J (eds) *Developing Focus Group Research.* London: Sage.

Middleton, R, Moloney T, Jackson, C, and Germains, R (2021) Education models embedding PD philosophy, values and impact – using the workplace as the main resource for learning, developing and improving (Chapter 6), in Kim Manley, et al. (eds) *International Practice Development in Health and Social Care.* John Wiley & Sons, Incorporated.

Miles, MB and Huberman, AM (1994) *Qualitative Data Analysis: An Expanded Sourcebook* (2nd edition). London: Sage.

Moher, D, Hopewell, S, Schulz, KF, Montori, V, Gøtzsche, PC, Devereaux, PJ, Elbourne, D, Egger, M and Altman, DG, for the CONSORT Group (2010) CONSORT 2010. Explanation and elaboration: updated guidelines for reporting parallel group randomised trial. *BMJ, 340*: c869.

Moule, P (2020) *Making Sense of Research in Nursing, Health and Social Care* (7th edition). London: Sage.

Moule, P and Goodman, M (2016) *Nursing Research: An Introduction* (3rd edition). London: Sage.

Muir Gray, JA (2009) *Evidence-Based Health Care: How to Make Health Policy and Management Decisions* (3rd edition). London: Churchill Livingstone.

Mulrow, CD (1995) Rationale for systematic reviews (Chapter 1), in Chalmers, I and Altman, DG (eds) *Systematic Reviews.* London: BMJ Publishing Group.

Myhre, J, Saga, S, Malmedal, W et al. (2020) Elder abuse and neglect: an overlooked patient safety issue. A focus group study of nursing home leaders' perceptions of elder abuse and neglect. *BMC Health Serv Res, 20*: 199. https://doi.org/10.1186/s12913-020-5047-4

Nardi, PM (2018) *Doing Survey Research: A Guide to Quantitative Methods* (4th edition). Boston, MA: Allyn & Bacon.

National Collaborating Centre for Methods and Tools (2011) *PARiHS Framework for Implementing Research into Practice.* Hamilton, ON: McMaster University. Available online at www.nccmt.ca/knowledge-repositories/search/85 (15 Feb 2024).

National Institute for Health and Care Excellence (NICE) (2009) *The Guidelines Manual 2009.* Available online at www.nice.org.uk/aboutnice/howwework/developing niceclinicalguidelines/clinicalguidelinedevelopmentmethods/GuidelinesManual2009. jsp (15 Feb 2024).

National Institute for Health and Care Excellence (NICE) (2014) *Safe Staffing for Nursing in Adult Inpatient Wards in Acute Hospitals (SG1).* Available online at www.nice.org.uk/guidance/sg1 (15 Feb 2024).

National Institute for Health and Care Excellence (NICE) (2016) *Development of a Safe Staffing App.* Available online at www.nice.org.uk/sharedlearning/development-of-a-safe-staffing-app (15 Feb 2024).

National Patient Safety Agency (NPSA) (2010) *Defining Research.* Available online at https://www.npsa.org.uk/ (15 Feb 2024).

Neuman, WL (2014) *Basics of Social Research: Qualitative and Quantitative Approaches* (3rd edition). Boston, MA: Allyn & Bacon.

NHS Centre for Reviews and Dissemination (2006) *Undertaking Systematic Reviews of Research on Effectiveness, CRD Report 4.* York: The University of York NHS Centre for Reviews and Dissemination.

NHS Improvement (2012) First steps towards quality improvement: a simple guide to improving services. Available online at www.slideshare.net/NHSImprovement/first-steps-towards-quality-improvement-a-simple-guide-to-improving-services (15 Feb 2024).

Nuremberg Code (1949) *Trials of War Criminals Before the Nuremberg Military Tribunals under Control Council Law No. 10,* Vol. 2, pp. 181–2. Washington, DC: US Government Printing Office. Available online at https://tile.loc.gov/storage-services/service/ll/llmlp/2011525364_NT_war-criminals_Vol-VI/2011525364_NT_war-criminals_Vol-VI. pdf (15 Feb 2024).

Nursing and Midwifery Council (NMC) (2018a) *Standards of Proficiency for Registered Nurses.* London: NMC.

Nursing and Midwifery Council (NMC) (2018b) *The Code: Professional Standards of Practice and Behaviour for Nurses, Midwives and Nursing Associates.* London: NMC.

O'Connor, T, Heron, J, Golding, J, Beveridge, M and Glover, V (2002) Maternal antenatal anxiety and children's behavioural/emotional problems at 4 years: report from the Avon Longitudinal Study of Parents and Children. *British Journal of Psychiatry, 180* (6): 502–8, doi:10.1192/bjp.180.6.502.

O'Leary, Z (2021) *The Essential Guide to Doing Your Research Project* (4th edition). London: Sage.

Parahoo, K (2014) *Nursing Research: Principles, Process and Issues* (3rd edition). Basingstoke: Palgrave Macmillan.

Parker, I (1992) *Discourse Dynamics: Critical Analysis for Social and Individual Psychology.* London: Routledge.

Parton, N (2004) From Maria Colwell to Victoria Climbié: reflections on public inquiries into child abuse a generation apart. *Child Abuse Review, 13*: 80–94.

Payne, G and Payne, J (2004) *Key Concepts in Social Research.* London: Sage.

Peat, J (2002) *Health Science Research: A Handbook of Quantitative Methods.* London: Sage.

Perkins, GD, Ji, C, Deakin, CD, Quinn, T, Nolan, JP, Scomparin, C, Regan, S, Long, J, Slowther, A, Pocock, H, Black, JJM, Moore, F, Fothergill, RT, Rees, N, O'Shea, L, Docherty, M, Gunson, I, Han, K, Charlton, K, Finn, J, Petrou, S, Stallard, N, Gates, S and Lall, R (2018) A randomized trial of epinephrine in out-of-hospital cardiac arrest. *New England Journal of Medicine, 379* (8): 711–721.

Philo, G (ed.) (1996) *Media and Mental Distress.* Harlow: Longman.

Potter, J and Wetherell, M (1987) *Discourse and Social Psychology: Beyond Attitudes and Behaviour.* London: Sage.

Powell, CV, Kelly, A-M and Williams, A (2001) Determining the minimum clinically significant difference in visual analog pain score for children. *Annals of Emergency Medicine, 37*: 28–31.

Pulido-Martos, M, Augusto-Landa, J and Lopez-Zafra, E (2012) Sources of stress in nursing students: a systematic review of quantitative studies. *International Nursing Review, 59*: 15–25.

Punch, K (2014) *Introduction to Social Research: Quantitative and Qualitative Approaches* (3rd edition). London: Sage.

Qiao, D, Whittaker, A and Tong, Z (2018) Media coverage, public awareness and state intervention in child abuse in China: an analysis of high profile cases. *Child Abuse Review, 27* (5): 378–88.

Quality Assurance Agency (QAA) (2001) *Code of Practice for the Assurance of Academic Quality and Standards in Higher Education: Placement Learning.* London: QAA.

Quinn, BL and Fantasia, HC (2018) Forming focus groups for pediatric pain research in nursing: a review of methods. *Pain Management Nursing, 19* (3): 303–12.

Riessman, C (2007) *Narrative Methods for the Human Sciences.* London: Sage.

Ring, N, Ritchie, K, Mandava, L and Jepson, R (2011) *A Guide to Synthesising Qualitative Research for Researchers Undertaking Health Technology Assessments and Systematic Reviews.* Glasgow: NHS Quality Improvement Scotland (NHS QIS).

Roberts, D and Dalziel, SR (2006) Antenatal corticosteroids for accelerating fetal lung maturation for women at risk of preterm birth. *Cochrane Database of Systematic Reviews, 3*: No.: CD004454, doi:10.1002/14651858.CD004454.pub2.

Robinson, FP (1970) *Effective Study* (4th edition). New York: Harper and Row.

Robson, C (2016) *Real World Research* (4th edition). Oxford: Blackwell.

Sackett, DL, Rosen, WMC, Gray, JAM and Richardson, WS (1996) Evidence-based medicine: what it is and what it isn't. *BMJ, 312*: 71–2.

Sackett, DL, Strauss, SE, Richardson, WS, Rosenberg, W and Haynes, RB (1997) *Evidence Based Medicine: How to Practise and Teach EBM*. Oxford: Churchill Livingstone.

Sarantakos, S (2013) *Social Research* (4th edition). Basingstoke: Palgrave Macmillan.

Saussure, F de (1983) *Course in General Linguistics*. London: Duckworth.

Scott, J (1990) *A Matter of Record: Documentary Sources in Social Research*. Cambridge: Polity Press.

Sharp, J (2009) *Success with Your Education Research Project*. Exeter: Learning Matters.

Silverman, D (2016) *Qualitative Research: Theory, Method and Practice* (4th edition). London: Sage.

Silverman, D (2017) *Doing Qualitative Research* (5th edition). London: Sage.

Smith, J, Pearson, L and Adams, J (2014) Incorporating a service improvement project into an undergraduate nursing programme: a pilot study. *International Journal of Nursing Practice, 20* (6): 623–628, doi: 10.1111/ijn.12217.

Strauss, A and Corbin, J (1998) *Basics of Qualitative Research: Techniques and Procedures for Developing Grounded Theory*. London: Sage.

Thurlow-Brown, N (1988) The Curate's Egg. Unpublished conference paper, North East Essex Mental Health Trust.

Tilling, K, Sterne, J, Brookes, S and Peters, TN (2005) Features and designs of randomized controlled trials and non-randomized experimental designs (Chapter 5), in Bowling, A and Ebrahim, S (eds) *Handbook of Health Research Methods: Investigation, Measurement and Analysis*. Milton Keynes: Open University Press.

Walliman, N (2016) *Social Research Methods* (2nd edition). London: Sage.

Walter, T (1996) A new model of grief: bereavement and biography, *Mortality, 1*:1, 7–25, doi:10.1080/713685822.

Waterman, H, Tillen, D, Dickson, R and de Koning, K (2001) Action research: a systematic review and guidance for assessment. *Health Technology Assessment, 5* (23): iii–157.

Whittaker, A, Densley, J, Cheston, L, Tyrell, T Higgins, M, Felix-Baptiste, C and Havard, T (2020) Reluctant Gangsters Revisited : The Evolution of Gangs from Postcodes to Profits. *European Journal of Criminal Policy and Research, 26*, 1–22. doi:10.1007/s10610-019-09408-4.

Williams, SJ and Caley, L (2020) *Improving Healthcare Services: Coproduction, Codesign and Operations*, Springer International Publishing AG.

Williamson, GR (2001) Does nursing need an ethical code for research? *NT Research,* *6* (4): 785–9.

Williamson, GR (2003) Misrepresenting random sampling? A systematic review of research papers in the *Journal of Advanced Nursing. Journal of Advanced Nursing, 44* (3): 278–88.

Williamson, GR and Prosser, S (2002) Action research: politics, ethics and participation. *Journal of Advanced Nursing, 40* (5): 587–93.

Williamson, GR, Collinson, S and Withers, N (2007) Patient satisfaction audit of a nurse-led lung cancer follow-up clinic. *Cancer Nursing Practice, 6* (8): 31–5.

Williamson, GR, Callaghan, L, Whittlesea, E and Heath, V (2010a) Improving student support using placement development teams: staff and student perceptions. *Journal of Clinical Nursing, 20*: 828–36.

Williamson, GR, Jenkinson, T and Proctor-Childs, T (2010b) *Contexts of Contemporary Nursing* (2nd edition). Exeter: Learning Matters.

Williamson, GR, Bellman, L and Webster, J (2012) *Action Research in Nursing and Healthcare.* London: Sage.

Williamson, GR, O'Connor, A, Chamberlain, C and Halpin, D (2018) mHealth resources for asthma and pregnancy care: methodological issues and social media recruitment. A discussion paper. *Journal of Advanced Nursing, 74*: 2442–9, doi:10.1111/jan.13773.

Williamson, GR, Kane, A, Plowright, H, Bunce, J, Clarke, D and Jamison, C, 2020. 'Thinking like a nurse'. Changing the culture of nursing students' clinical learning: Implementing collaborative learning in practice. *Nurse Education in Practice, 43*, 102742.

Willis Commission (2012) *Quality with Compassion: The Future of Nursing Education.* Report of the Willis Commission on Nursing Education. London: Royal College of Nursing.

Wills, J, Whittaker, A, Rickard, W and Felix, C (2017) Troubled, troubling or in trouble: the stories of troubled families. *British Journal of Social Work, 47* (4): 989–1006.

Wong, PTP (2002) *How to Write a Research Proposal.* Available online at www.drpaulwong.com/how-to-write-a-research-proposal/ (15 Feb 2024).

World Medical Association (2013) Declaration of Helsinki: ethical principles for medical research involving human subjects. *Journal of the American Medical Association, 310* (20): 2191–4.

Yin, R (2018) *Case Study Research: Design and Methods* (6th edition). London: Sage.

Yost, J, Thompson, D, Ganann, R, Aloweni, F, Newman, K, McKibbon, A, Dobbins, M and Ciliska, D (2014) Knowledge translation strategies for enhancing nurses' evidence-informed decision making: a scoping review. *Worldviews on Evidence-Based Nursing, 11* (3): 156–67, doi:10.1111/wvn.12043.

Index

Note: References in *italics* are to figures, those in **bold** to tables; 'g' refers to the Glossary